This book is due for return on or before the last date shown below.

Handbook of Vitreo-Retinal Disorder Management

A Practical Reference Guide

Handbook of Vitreo-Retinal Disorder Management

A Practical Reference Guide

Susanna S Park

University of California Davis, USA

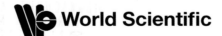

NEW JERSEY • LONDON • SINGAPORE • BEIJING • SHANGHAI • HONG KONG • TAIPEI • CHENNAI

Published by

World Scientific Publishing Co. Pte. Ltd.
5 Toh Tuck Link, Singapore 596224
USA office: 27 Warren Street, Suite 401-402, Hackensack, NJ 07601
UK office: 57 Shelton Street, Covent Garden, London WC2H 9HE

Library of Congress Cataloging-in-Publication Data
Handbook of vitreo-retinal disorder management : a practical reference guide / [edited by]
Susanna S. Park.
    p. ; cm.
  Includes bibliographical references and index.
  ISBN 978-9814663298 (hardcover : alk. paper)
  I. Park, Susanna S., editor.
  [DNLM: 1. Retinal Diseases--therapy--Atlases. 2. Retinal Diseases--therapy--Handbooks.
3. Diagnostic Techniques, Ophthalmological--Atlases. 4. Diagnostic Techniques,
Ophthalmological--Handbooks. 5. Retinal Diseases--diagnosis--Atlases. 6. Retinal Diseases--
diagnosis--Handbooks. WW 39]
  RE551
  617.7'35--dc23
                                                                    2015013708

British Library Cataloguing-in-Publication Data
A catalogue record for this book is available from the British Library.

Typeset by Stallion Press
Email: enquires@stallionpress.com

Printed in Singapore

Preface

This handbook was written to provide a concise, affordable quick reference book for practicing ophthalmologists and vitreo-retinal specialists on the latest recommendations regarding the management of common vitreo-retinal disorders seen in everyday clinical practice. Although some of the information included in this handbook may appear geared toward retinal specialists, we hope that all eye care providers will find this handbook helpful in treating and educating patients with common retinal disorders. The information is provided in outline form for conciseness and easy-reading. Abbreviations are sometimes used, and an appendix of abbreviations is provided at the end of the book for reference. In order to keep the information limited to one volume, my contributing authors and I chose to include only the most important information that clinicians will need in diagnosing and managing patients with common vitreo-retinal conditions. This book does not provide a comprehensive overview of every vitreo-retinal disorder. A list of references is provided at the end of each chapter for further reading, and figures are included to illustrate representative diagnostic findings.

With the recent rapid advances in new diagnostic tools and therapies, there are many more options we can offer to our patients with retinal problems. This is a wonderful time to be treating our patients with retinal conditions, but it can be a confusing time. The goal of this book is to summarize the available options and provide a roadmap for the clinicians based on the latest reported findings. When applicable, the pros and cons of various treatments are included. Since medicine is often an "art" rather than a "science," the recommendations outlined in this handbook may not be universally shared by practicing retinal specialists. Furthermore, new treatments may be in development, even as we write this book, that may change the way we practice in a few years. Nonetheless, my contributing authors and I have tried our best to present the most current and universally accepted practice guidelines. In doing so, it was a great pleasure for me to work with vitreo-retinal fellows and colleagues at our home institution and nationally to produce this first handbook. I learned as much from my fellow contributing authors as I did preparing my portion of the writing. We hope the readers also find this handbook as informative and useful.

Susanna S. Park MD, PhD
Contributing Author and Editor

Contributing Authors

1. David R.P. Almeida MD, MBA, PhD
    Vitreo-retinal Surgical Fellow
    Department of Ophthalmology
    University of Iowa School of Medicine
    Iowa City, IA

2. Antonio Capone Jr., MD
    Professor of Ophthalmology
    Associated Retinal Consultants
    William Beaumont Hospital
    Royal Oak, MI

3. Eric K. Chin, MD
    Vitreo-retinal Surgical Fellow
    Department of Ophthalmology School of Medicine
    University of Iowa School of Medicine
    Iowa City, IA

4. Kimberly A. Drenser, MD, PhD
    Associate Professor of Ophthalmology
    Associated Retinal Consultants
    William Beaumont Hospital
    Royal Oak, MI

5. Jonathan Kim, MD
   Director, Ocular Oncology
   A. Linn Murphree Chair in Retinoblastoma
   Associate Professor of Ophthalmology
   Children's Hospital Los Angeles
   USC Keck School of Medicine
   Los Angeles, CA

6. Elad Moisseiev, MD
   Vitreo-retinal Surgical Fellow
   University of California Davis Eye Center
   Sacramento, CA

7. Ala Moshiri, MD, PhD
   Assistant Professor of Ophthalmology
   Vitreo-retinal Service
   Department of Ophthalmology & Vision Science
   University of California Davis Eye Center
   Sacramento, CA

8. Bobeck Modjtahedi, MD
   Vitreoretinal Surgical Fellow
   Massachusetts Eye and Ear Infirmary
   Harvard Medical School
   Boston, MA

9. Lawrence S. Morse, MD, PhD
   Professor of Ophthalmology
   Director of Vitreoretinal Service
   Department of Ophthalmology & Vision Science
   University of California Davis Eye Center
   Sacramento, CA

10. Senad Osmanovic, MD
    Vitreoretinal Surgical Fellow
    Department of Ophthalmology & Vision Science
    University of California Davis Eye Center
    Sacramento, CA

11. Susanna S. Park, MD, PhD
     Professor of Ophthalmology
     Director of Vitreo-retinal Fellowship
     Director of Ocular Oncology
     Vitreo-retinal Service
     Department of Ophthalmology & Vision Science
     University of California Davis Eye Center
     Sacramento, CA

12. Amar Patel, MD
     Vitreoretinal Specialist/ Staff Surgeon
     The Permanente Medical Group, Inc.
     Oakland, CA

13. Suma P. Shankar, MD, PhD
     Assistant Professor
     Department of Human Genetics &
     Department of Ophthalmology
     Medical Consultant, Emory Genetics Laboratory
     Emory University School of Medicine
     Decatur, GA

14. Sumeer Thinda, MD
     Vitreoretinal Surgical Fellow
     Department of Ophthalmology & Vision Science
     University of California Davis Eye Center
     Sacramento, CA

15. Benjamin J. Thomas, MD
     Vitreoretinal Surgical Fellow
     Associated Retinal Consultants
     William Beaumont Hospital
     Royal Oak, MI

16. Michael T. Trese, MD
     Professor of Ophthalmology
     Associated Retinal Consultants
     William Beaumont Hospital
     Royal Oak, MI

17. Gary Yau, MD
Senior Ophthalmology Resident
Department of Ophthalmology
Queen's University
Kingston, Ontario, Canada

18. Glenn Yiu, MD, PhD
Assistant Professor of Ophthalmology
Vitreo-retinal Service
Department of Ophthalmology & Vision Science
University of California Davis Eye Center
Sacramento, CA

19. Yoshihiro Yonekawa, MD
Vitreoretinal Surgical Fellow
Associated Retinal Consultants
William Beaumont Hospital
Royal Oak, MI

Contents

SECTION 1:
DIAGNOSTIC TESTING

Chapter 1: Retinal Imaging

Amar Patel and Susanna S. Park

1. Optical Coherence Tomography (OCT)

a. Non-invasive real-time cross-sectional imaging
b. Specifications (see Table 1 for various types of OCT)

    i. Axial resolutions variable depending on type of OCT
    ii. Transverse resolution 10 to 20 μm
    iii. Macular scans are typically 6 mm × 6 mm

c. Normal macular morphology on OCT (Figure 1A)

    i. The interface between the posterior hyaloid and the internal limiting membrane is visualized when the hyaloid is separated from retina.
    ii. The fovea is thinned due to the absence of the inner retinal layers. The ellipsoid zone, also called the inner segment-outer segment junction (IS/OS), is elevated slightly due to the presence of densely packed cones in the foveal center

Table 1. Comparison of OCT modalities.

OCT Modality	Time Domain	Spectral Domain	Swept Source
Laser source	~800 nm	~800 nm	1050 nm
A-Scan speed	400/sec	25,000–50,000/sec	200,000/sec
Axial resolution	8–10 μm	5–7 μm	5–7 μm
Structures imaged	Retina	Retina	Retina and Choroid

iii. Reflectivity of retinal layers is based upon the arrangement of their structures as well as their biological densities and degree of pigmentation

1. High reflectivity: the nerve fiber layer (NFL), the inner plexiform layer (IPL), and outer plexiform layer (OPL) are highly reflective due to the horizontally oriented axonal structures. The retinal pigment epithelium (RPE) and choriocapillaris form the outermost highly reflective structure visible due to their high melanin and vascular content, respectively

2. Lower reflectivity: the ganglion cell layer (GCL), the inner nuclear layer (INL), and the outer nuclear layer (ONL) are less reflective due to the vertical orientation of their elements

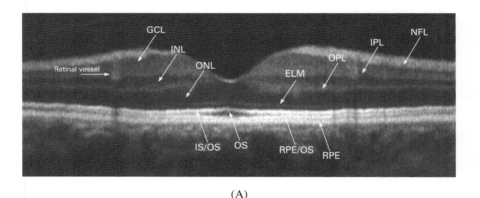

(A)

Figure 1.   Spectral-domain OCT.

(A) B-scan image of a normal macula showing the various retinal layers; nerve fiber layer (NFL), ganglion cell layer (GCL), inner plexiform layer (IPL), inner nuclear layer (INL), outer plexiform layer (OPL), outer nuclear layer (ONL), external limiting membrane (ELM), and retinal pigment epithelium (RPE). (B) A commercial spectral-domain OCT (Cirrus, Zeiss) showing diffuse macular thinning (yellow-red zones in the ETDRS thickness map and blue in the macular cube volume scan) in an eye with exudative macular degeneration following anti-VEGF therapy. No residual macular fluid is detected but a residual sub macular hyperreflective lesion is noted. The macular cube scan (right) shows the three-dimensional depiction of regional changes in the macula at various layers. Image signal strength is denoted at the top of the page.

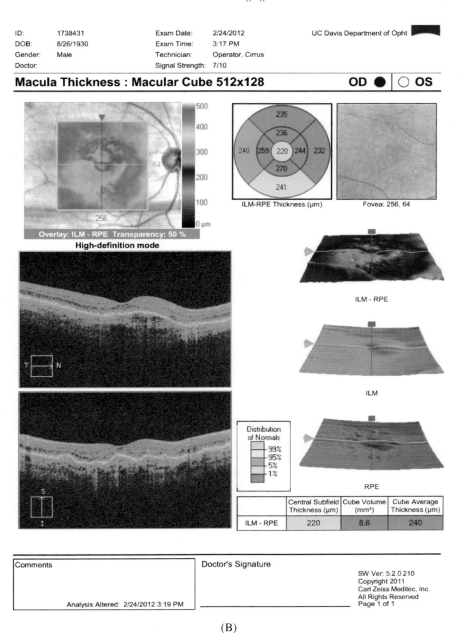

(B)

Figure 1. (*Continued*)

d. Image orientation and quality

    i. Scanned images have a legend that indicates the directionality of the currently displayed scan. By convention, the right side of the image corresponds to the arrowhead

    ii. Signal-to-noise ratio is displayed and labeled as signal strength. (Figure 1B) A signal strength of 10 represents the highest quality imaging, whereas a signal strength of zero represents the lowest quality. Signal strength can be affected by media opacities. Adequate signal strength is ≥5

    iii. For macular thickness measurements, ILM and RPE borders are corrected by automated algorithm. However, manual correction option is available

    iv. Macula centered in the scan: The foveal depression should be in the center of the scan

e. Macular thickness map (Figure 1B)

    i. The macula is artificially divided into nine regions of the ETDRS macular thickness map and the average retinal thickness is calculated for each region. The inner circle of the map has a diameter of 1.0 mm and correlates roughly with the fovea. The middle circle has a diameter of 3.0 mm and the outer circle a diameter of 6.0 mm, which is the length of the axial scans. A color coding system is used to correlate the thickness to the normative values. Pink denotes >99% normal, green denotes 95% normal, and red denotes <1% normal

    ii. A color coded macular thickness map of the three-dimensional reconstruction of the entire macula image (macular cube) is also available along with a legend displayed to facilitate rapid interpretation of the numerical values. Greater retinal thickness is represented by the "hotter" colors such as red and white. Average retinal thickness is represented by green, thin and atrophic areas of retina are represented by the "cooler" colors such as blue or black

    iii. Central retinal or foveal thickness and total volume of the macula are displayed in numerical format

f. Choroidal imaging: the choriocapillaris and the deeper larger sized choroidal vessels cannot be seen well using conventional OCT due to the shadowing from the overlying RPE. The following modalities are useful for imaging the choroid

    i. Enhanced depth imaging (EDI)-OCT

        1. Place the objective lens of the device closer to the eye so that an inverted image is obtained. This maneuver allows deeper structures to be placed closer to the zero delay, thereby allowing for better visualization of the choroid

ii. Swept source

    1. Sweeps a narrow bandwidth laser with longer wavelength (1,050 nm) through a broad optical spectrum and detects back-scattered intensity with a photodetector. Its faster speed with increased resolution allows for faster and more accurate images of the retina and choroid (Figure 2)

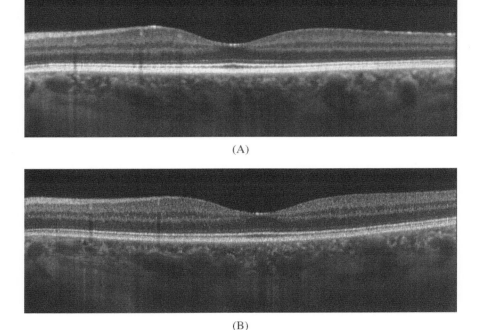

(A)

(B)

Figure 2. Enhanced depth imaging (EDI) OCT images of the retina and choroid: spectral-domain versus swept-source OCT. (A) Research-grade high resolution spectral-domain OCT using EDI mode shows good resolution of both the retinal and choroidal layers in the macula of this normal subject. (B) Research-grade high resolution swept-source OCT using EDI mode image of the same subject showed improved resolution of both the retinal and choroidal layers when compared to images obtained using spectral-domain OCT. In both images the choroidal layer is better visualized than in Figure 1 using normal mode OCT imaging. (Images courtesy of the Advanced Retinal Imaging Laboratory at the University of California Davis Eye Center, Sacramento, CA.)

2. Fluorescein Angiography (FA)

a. Fluorescein sodium, intravenous dye

   i. Synthesized from the petroleum derivatives resorcinol and phthalic anhydride

   ii. The wavelengths used to excite the fluorescein molecules range from 465–490 nm (blue light). The excited molecules produce yellow-green fluorescent light, with a wavelength of between 520–530 nm that is captured with the camera

   iii. Up to 70–80% of the injected dye molecules are bound mostly to serum albumin leaving an unbound portion that can diffuse through small intercellular spaces which is detected angiographically

   iv. Removed from the systemic circulation via the kidneys and liver

   v. Side effects:

      1. Yellowing of the skin and conjunctiva (up to 6–12 hours)
      2. Orange-yellow discoloration of the urine (24–36 hours)
      3. Nausea, vomiting, or vasovagal reactions (10%)
      4. Urticaria (1%)
      5. Anaphylactic reactions (1 in 100,000)

b. Blood-retinal Barriers

   i. Inner retina: tight junctions are present throughout the retinal vasculature, preventing fluorescein dye to leak into the surrounding tissue

   ii. Outer retina and choriod: vessels within the choriocapillaris have large fenestrations allowing free fluorescein molecules to quickly leak out into the surrounding choroidal tissue. The retinal pigment epithelial is a monocellular layer of cells connected by tight junctions. These junctions prevent leakage of fluorescein from the choroid to the sensory retina and also acts like an optical filter blocking the background of the choroidal fluorescence

c. Normal Fluorescein

   i. Red Free Image (Green Filter): pre-injection

      1. Green light is also absorbed by blood, but is partially reflected by the retinal pigmentation
      2. Green light enhances the visibility of the retinal vasculature, and common findings such as hemorrhages, drusen and exudates. Visualization of some retinal surface changes also may be enhanced

ii. Choroidal Flush (Figure 3A)

    1. The choriocapillaries quickly fills with dye in about 10–15 seconds after injection

    2. A patchy, lobular choroidal pattern or choroidal flush is observed

    3. Perfusion of any cilioretinal arteries (present in 20% of population) occurs simultaneously with that of the choroidal vessels

iii. Arterial Phase (Figure 3B)

    1. Central retinal artery begins to fill in 1–3 seconds after the choroidal flush

    2. Within seconds, the entire arterial side of the retinal vasculature is filled with fluorescein dye, marking the end of the arterial phase of the study

iv. Arteriovenous or Laminar Venous Phase (Figure 3C)

    1. Retinal venules fill within 5–10 seconds

    2. Perifoveal capillary network is best visualized. The normal foveal avascular zone is 400–500 microns in size

v. Venous Phase (Figure 3D)

    1. Venous columns become wider within 5–15 seconds until the entire venous lumen fills with dye (usually by 34 seconds following dye injection)

    2. Filling progresses from the venous wall inward towards the central lumen because the blood velocity is slowest near the wall and fastest at the center of the vessel

vi. Late Phase (Figure 3E)

    1. Recirculation phase starts beyond 30 seconds

    2. Late frames show fluorescence of the choroid and sclera (the large amount of dye in the extravascular spaces and sclera, causes the larger choroidal vessels to appear hypo fluorescent)

    3. Fluorescence of the optic disc may be seen primarily, caused by staining of the lamina cribrosa

d. Abnormal Fluorescence

  i. Causes of hypofluorescence: see Figure 4

  ii. Causes of hyperfluorecence: see Figure 5

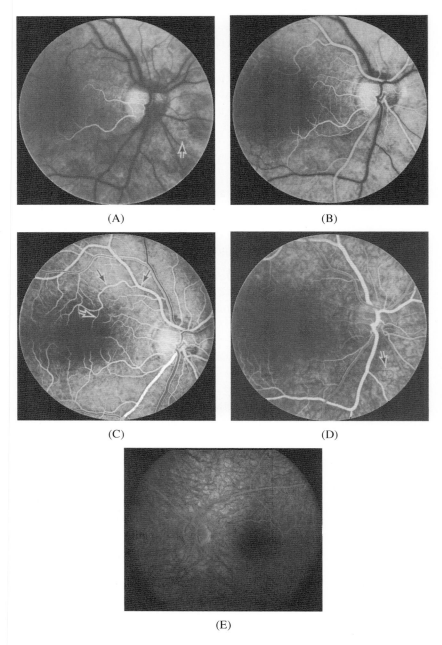

(A)   (B)

(C)   (D)

(E)

Figure 3. Normal fluorescein angiography; (A) choroidal flush, (B) arterial phase, (C) arteriovenous phase, (D) venous phase, (E) late phase.

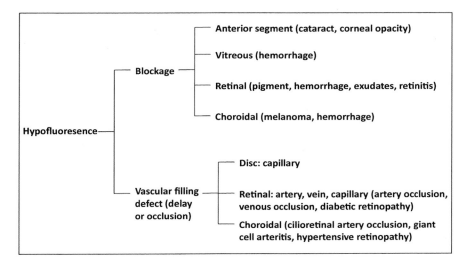

Figure 4. Diagram of abnormal hypofluoresence in fluorescein angiography.

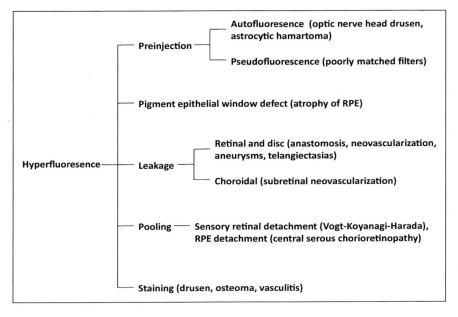

Figure 5. Diagram of abnormal hyperfluoresence in fluorescein angiography.

3. Indocyanine Green (ICG) Angiography

a. ICG dye

    i. About 98% of dye is bound to serum protein, such that, there is less leakage and reduced passage through choroidal fenestrations. This allows enhanced imaging of choroidal vessels and choroidal lesions (Figure 6)

    ii. Absorption is in near-infrared (805 nm) with emission in infrared (835 nm). Since the RPE and choroid absorb 60–75% of the blue green light used in FA (500 nm) and only 20–38% of the near infrared light (800 nm) used in ICG angiography, ICG dye results in improved visualization through pigment (melanin, xanthophyll), thin layers of hemorrhage, lipid exudates, and serosanguineous fluid

    iii. Adverse reactions:

        1. Contains 5% iodine, therefore should be used with caution in patients with iodine or shellfish allergy

        2. Should be avoided in uremic patients with liver disease where delayed clearance has been reported

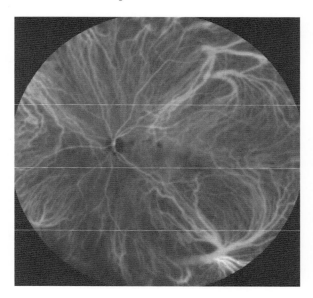

Figure 6. Indocyanine green (ICG) angiogram. This wide angle image of the left eye of a patient with old chorioretinitis, demonstrates the improved visualization of the choroidal circulation using this dye when compared to fluorescein angiography. Small focal hypofluorescence spots in the macula may represent focal choroidal filling defects.

b. Normal ICG Angiogram

   i. Early phase (2 seconds to 5 minutes)

      1. Hypo fluorescent optic disc (watershed zone)
      2. Prominent filling choroidal arteries and early choroidal vein filling

   ii. Early middle-phase (5 minutes)

      1. Watershed zone fills
      2. Choroidal arteries fade and choroidal veins fill.

   iii. Late middle-phase (15 minutes)

      1. Choroidal vessels fade
      2. Diffuse hyper fluorescence as dye diffuses from choriocapillaris
      3. Hyper fluorescent lesions appear

   iv. Late phase (>15 minutes)

      1. Hypo fluorescence of large choroidal vessels against background of hyper fluorescence
      2. Retinal vessels are not visible

c. Abnormal ICG: causes of abnormal ICG fluorescence are summarized in Figure 7

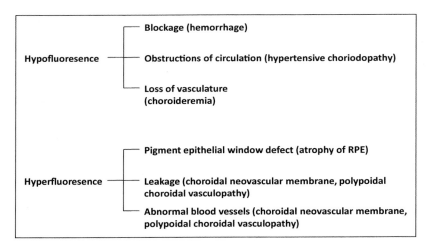

Figure 7. Diagram of abnormal fluoresence in indocyanine green angiography.

4. Fundus Autofluoresence (AF)

a. Fundus AF

    i.   Lipofuscin is a byproduct of photoreceptor outer segment phagocytosis that accumulates in RPE, which is an indirect marker of metabolic activity

    ii. Excited by a short wavelength light (488 nm), RPE lipofuscin granules emit a longer wavelength (500–750 nm)

b. Normal fundus AF image

    i.   Disk: no AF since no RPE
    ii.   Vessels: decreased AF due to masking of RPE by overlying blood.
    iii. Fovea: decreased AF due to absorption of short wavelength light by melanin and luteal pigment in central macula
    iv.   Parafoveal area: increased AF
    v.   Periphery: decreased AF

c. Abnormal fundus AF

    i.   Decreased of absent AF: reduced metabolic demand due to photoreceptor cell death with or without RPE atrophy or disruption of the retinoid cycle

         Examples: geographic atrophy, Chronic central serous chorioretinopathy, Multiple evanescent white dot syndrome

    ii. Increased AF: increased lipofuscin accumulation from disrupted RPE phagocytic function or an inability of the RPE to recycle metabolites

         Example: flecks of Stargardt's disease/fundus flavimaculatus, RPE surrounding areas of atrophy or photoreceptor disruption such as in cone dystrophy, adjacent to areas of atrophy in maculopathy associated with mitochondrial mutations and the vitelliform material in pattern dystrophy, Best's disease

References

Alam S, Zawadrzki RJ, Choi S, *et al*. Clinical applications of rapid serial fourier domain optical coherence tomography for macular mapping. *Ophthalmology* 2006;113:1425–1431.

Chinn SR, Swanson EA, Fujimoto JG. Optical coherence tomography using a frequency-tunable optical source. *Opt Lett* 1997;22(5):340–342.

Hirata M, Tsujikawa A, Matsumoto A, *et al*. Macular choroidal thickness and volume in normal subjects measured by swept-source optical coherence tomography. *Invest Ophthalmol Vis Sci* 2011;52:4971–4978.

Schmitz-Valckenberg S, Holz FG, Bird AC, *et al*. Fundus autofluoresence imaging: review and perspectives. *Retina* 2008;28(3):385–409.

Spaide RF, Koisumi H, Posonni MC. Enhanced depth imaging spectral-domain optical coherence tomography. *Am J Ophthalmol* 2008;146:496–500.

Chapter 2: Electroretinography

Amar Patel and Ala Moshiri

1. Electroretinogram (ERG)

a. Electrical response of the eye that originates from extracellular currents that are generated in response to a light stimulus
b. Components of the ERG signal (Table 1 and Figure 1)

    i. a wave: photoreceptor cell bodies

        1. Initial negative wave-form
        2. Light absorbance by the visual pigment molecules in the outer segments of the photoreceptors reduces the "dark" current and therefore, can be viewed as eliciting a "light" current. This current is expressed as a negative wave when recorded from the vitreous or the cornea

    ii. b wave: primarily bipolar cells, muller cell component

        1. First positive wave-form
        2. Reflects light-induced electrical activity in retinal cells post-synaptic to the photoreceptors

    iii. c wave: retinal pigment epithelium

        1. Second positive wave-form
        2. Depends upon the integrity of the photoreceptors because light absorption in the photoreceptors triggers the chain of events leading to the decrease in extracellular concentration of potassium ions
        3. Used to assess the functional integrity of the photoreceptors, the pigment epithelial cells and the interactions between them

Table 1. Diseases associated with abnormal ERG.

Normal a-wave, Reduced b-wave	Reduced a-wave and b-wave	Normal Photopic, Abnormal Scoptopic	Abnormal Photopic, Normal Scoptopic
Central retinal vein occlusion	Ophthalmic artery occlusion	Retinitis pigmentosa (early)	Cone dystrophy
Central retinal artery occlusion	Retinitis pigmentosa (late)	Congenital stationary night blindness	Stationary cone disorders (Achromatopsia, Blue cone monochromatism)
Congenital stationary night blindness	Hydroxychloroquine toxicity		
X-linked retinoschisis	Retinal detachment		

    iv. Early receptor potentials: outer segments of photoreceptors

        1. Appears immediately after stimulus onset and has a biphasic pattern

        2. Ends within 1.5 ms and is followed by the a-wave

        3. Follows the concentration of the visual pigment during light adaptation and in the dark, following an exposure to bright light, causes substantial pigment bleaching

        4. Estimate rhodopsin density in patients suffering from retinitis pigmentosa

    v. Oscillatory potential: inner plexiform layer (extracellular electrical currents between amacrine cells, ganglion cells and bipolar cells)

        1. Low amplitude oscillating waves on the rising phase of the b-wave of bright flash ERG

        2. Indicates mild retinal ischemia in the inner retina such as in diabetic retinopathy

        3. Assesses the balance between retinal metabolic needs and retinal vascular supply

c. Rod and cone system

    i. Rod system (night vision)

        1. Very sensitive to dim light stimuli in the dark-adapted state while under background illumination, it saturates and does not respond to light increment or decrement

ii. Cone system (day vision)

    1. Not as sensitive but is characterized by the ability to adapt to bright lights, processes that allow vision to adapt to background illumination over a wide range of intensities

d. State of adaptation

  i. Light Adaptation (photopic)

    1. Light stimulus is applied under background illumination that saturates the rod system

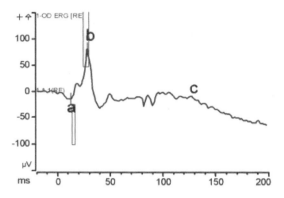

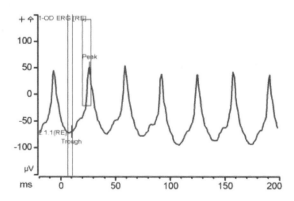

Figure 1. Full-field electroretinogram (ff ERG). A typical full-field ERG recording obtained under scotopic conditions. (Top) Full-field amplitude of light-adapted response. Flicker response amplitude. The rectangular boxes represent the range of age-matched normal amplitude values for each recording.

2. Small amplitude but of very fast kinetics; time to peak is about 30 to 32 ms
3. Reflects activity in the cone system
4. Flicker: poor response at 30 cycles/second indicates abnormal cone function

ii. Dark adaptation (scotopic)

1. Light stimulus is applied after the subject is kept in darkness for about 30 min, the ERG is of considerably larger amplitude (about 4 folds) and is characterized by slow temporal properties
2. Time to peak of the b-wave is about 60 ms
3. Mixed rod-cone response (the cone system is operational too) but mainly reflects the activity in the rod system since the cone system contribution is considerably smaller
4. Bright flash: measures maximal cone and rod response

2. Multifocal Electroretinogram

a. Tests the ERG from a localized defined part of the retina, usually centered on fixation with five concentric rings to test the function of the macula
b. Uses mathematical sequences called binary m-sequences and a program that can extract hundreds of focal ERGs from a single electrical signal
c. This system allows assessment of ERG activity in small areas of the retina
d. With this method one can record mf ERGs (multifocal elctroretinography) from hundreds of retinal areas in a few minutes
e. Small Scotomas in the retina can be mapped and degree of retinal dysfunction quantified.
f. ERG electrodes are used to record ERGs from the cornea of a dilated eye similar to full-field ERG. The recordings can be done during the same session as the full-field ERG
g. Useful to diagnose or screen for macular disease not obvious on clinical examination, such as macular degeneration, macular dystrophies, toxic maculopathies, etc.
h. The b-wave voltages from the patient are transformed into a color plot. Colors reflect standard deviations from age-matched normative data of average ERG amplitudes (Figure 2)
i. One of the best uses of mf ERGs is distinguishing between retinal and optic nerve etiology of visual problems in patients with no obvious fundus abnormalities. These types of patients can include OMD (occult macular dystrophy), AZOOR (acute zonal occult outer retinopathy), and others

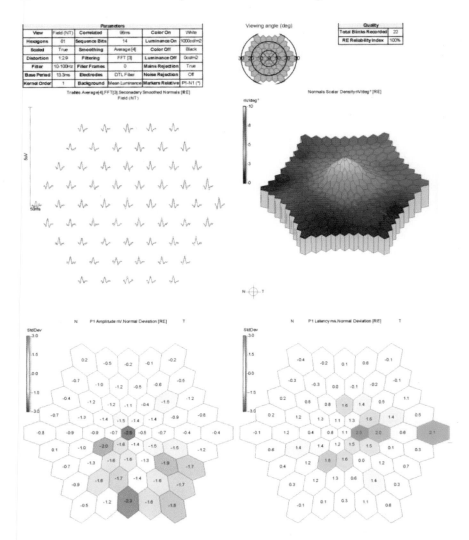

Figure 2.   mfERG. This mulifocal ERG of an eye with age-related macular degeneration shows some focal abnormalities in amplitude (red-pink hexogons in the lower left map) and latency (green hexagons in the lower right map).

References

1. McCulloch DL, Marmor MF, Brigell MG, *et al. Ophthalmol* 2014;
2. Hood DC, Bach M, Brigell M, *et al.* International society for clinical electrophysiology of vision. *Ophthalmol* 2012;124(1):1–13.
3. The Electroretinogram: ERG by Ido Perlman — Webvision Retrieved from http://webvision.med.utah.edu/book/electrophysiology/the-electroretinogram-erg/
4. The Electroretinogram and Electro-oculogram: Clinical Applications Retrieved from http://webvision.med.utah.edu/book/electrophysiology/the-electroretinogram-clinical-applications/

Chapter 3: Genetic Testing

Suma P. Shankar and Susanna S. Park

1. Advantages of Genetic Testing

- Increases the accuracy and specificity of the diagnosis
- Peace of mind for those with known family history of certain genetic conditions, if genetic test results are negative
- Potential participation in clinical trials including trials for gene therapy
- Increase our understanding of pathogenesis of the condition
- Avoid unnecessary screening tests. For example, examination under anesthesia for family members of retinoblastoma patients, if negative genetic test

2. Limitations of Genetic Testing

- Prone to errors as any other medical tests
- Results may take weeks to months to obtain
- Genetic testing is not a 100% sensitive or specific test. The results are graded in terms of pathogenic probability. A negative test result does not mean the patient does not have the clinical condition
- Genetic tests are expensive. They may not be covered by medical insurance
- Many inherited diseases may not have a gene identified as yet

3. American Academy of Ophthalmology Recommendations for Genetic Testing

- Recommend genetic testing only if clinical findings suggest a condition whose causative gene(s) have been identified: e.g. inherited retinal diseases, retinoblastoma, von Hippel–Lindau

- Use CLIA (Clinical Laboratory Improvement Amendments) — approved laboratories: http://www.ncbi.nlm.nih.gov/gtr/
- Provide a copy of the test result to the patient
- Encourage the involvement of a genetic counselor and/or physician for all genetic tests and discourage patients from obtaining direct-to-consumer genetic tests
- Avoid routine genetic testing for genetically complex disorders (e.g. age-related macular degeneration) unless specific treatment or surveillance strategies have been shown to be beneficial
- Testing of pre-symptomatic children less than 18 years of age for adult-onset diseases without cure is not recommended

4. Inherited Retinal Diseases (Refer to Section 4 for more details)

1. Introduction: inherited retinal diseases are a significant cause of visual morbidity, many of them presenting at birth or in early childhood. They are a genetically and phenotypically diverse group of dystrophies and degenerations. Clinical diagnosis is made based on clinical presentation, fundus appearance and/or photoreceptor dysfunctions identified by electrophysiological tests.

   Genetic testing allows for molecular diagnosis and over 221 genes causing retinal, choroidal and optic nerve diseases have been identified. Retinal dystrophies may be part of systemic conditions such as Bardet Beidl syndrome.

   Given the heterogeneity, a thorough clinical evaluation and a complete family history, including pedigree construction, are necessary to identify the mode of inheritance and in to order correct genetic tests.

2. Clinical Features

- Poor vision presentation ranging from birth to adulthood
- Congenital nystagmus
- Night vision problems
- Color vision problems
- Peripheral field loss
- Systemic features: polydactyly, brachydactyly, obesity, history of renal disease, neurological disease, or hypertension should be noted
- Fundus appearance may be normal as in Leber congenital amaurosis
- Optic nerve pallor, bone spicules, pigmentary clumping, changes, arteriolar narrowing, drusen and retinal pigment epithelium (RPE) and choroidal atrophy, cystoid macular edema as in retinitis pigmentosa
- Retinal flecks or yellow/white deposits as in fleck retinopathies

3. Initial Evaluation
   a. History

      Determine if congenital or new change in fundus appearance:

      1. Compare with any prior fundus photographs available
      2. Any associated visual symptoms — change in visual acuity, metamorphopsia, color vision problems, night vision and peripheral field loss
      3. Detailed family history information is crucial to determine the mode of inheritance in a patient and includes:

         (i) Autosomal dominant
         (ii) Autosomal recessive
         (iii) X-linked recessive
         (iv) Digenic inheritance
         (v) Mitochondrial mutations

         In sporadic cases without other known affected relatives, the mode of inheritance may be unclear

4. Review of systems: essential to evaluate for any syndromic associations with retinal dystrophies

   a. Eye Examination: document appearance of fundus
   b. Diagnostic Tests: baseline and serial follow-up for comparison

      i. Color fundus photography
      ii. Optical coherence tomography (OCT)
      iii. Electroretinogram (ERG), multifocal ERG
      iv. Goldman visual fields
      v. Fluorescein angiogram
      vi. Autofluorescence

5. Genetic testing

   a. Based on clinical diagnosis, several options for genetic testing are available

      i. **Single gene testing** is recommended for conditions such as Stargardt's disease where only one gene *ABCA4* is the most common etiology
      ii. **Targeted next generation sequencing panels and microarrays or aCGH (array comparitive genomic hybridization)** are recommended for conditions such as isolated retinitis pigmentosa where >50 different genes have been identified

iii. **Microarrays or aCGH (array comparitive genomic hybridiza-tion)** are recommended for conditions such as retinitis pigmentosa where >50 different genes have been identified.

iv. **Allele specific targeted testing** is recommended for identifying most common mutations as in Leber's hereditary optic neuropathy

b. *Exome and genome analysis is not recommended in retinal dystrophies given the possibility of incidental findings in many genes that are unrelated to the retinal condition, for example, in BRCA1 or 2, genes causing breast and other cancers may be found*

c. List of laboratories offering RP genetic testing: http://www.ncbi.nlm.nih. gov/gtr/labs/?term=retinitis+pigmentosa

d. The types of testing for retinal diseases that are genetically heterogeneous but phenotypically similar include *Next Generation sequencing and Deletion/Duplication Panels*. These should be comprehensive and targeted. Some examples of the targeted panels are described as follows:

Achromatopsia, Cone, and Cone-rod Dystrophy: This panel testing can be useful for individuals presenting with decreased central vision, photophobia, ERG finding of absent/decreased cone function. Causative genes include: *ABCA4, ADAM9, AIPL1, BEST1, C8orf37, CABP4, CACNA1F, CACNA2D4, CDHR1, CEP290, CERKL, CNGA3, CNGB3, CNNM4, CRX, GNAT2, GUCA1A, GUCA1B, GUCY2D, KCNV2, PAX6, PDE6C, PDE6H, PITPNM3, PROM1, PRPH2, RAX2, RBP4, RDH5, RGS9, RGS9BP, RIMS1, RPGR, RPGRIP1, SEMA4A, UNC119*

Congenital Stationary Night Blindness: Test to determine this condition may be recommended for individuals with myopia, night vision problems and decreased scotopic function and negative B wave on ERG but non-progressive. Causative genes include: *GNAT1, PDE6B, RHO, CABP4, GNAT1, GPR179, GRK1, GRM6, LRIT3, RDH5, SAG, SLC24A1, TRPM1, CACNA1F, NYX*

Leber Congenital Amaurosis: This condition may be present in individuals who have suffered vision loss since birth, with almost normal appearing retina and non-recordable ERG. Causative genes include: *CRX, IMPDH1, OTX2, AIPL1, CABP4, CEP290, CRB1, CRX, DTHD1, GDF6, GUCY2D, IQCB1, KCNJ13, LCA5, LRAT, NMNAT1, RD3, RDH12, RPE65, RPGRIP1, SPATA7, TULP1*

Macular Dystrophy, Degeneration, Stargardt Disease: This disease will present in individuals with flecks, pigmentary changes, and/or lipofuscin-like deposits in the macula with normal ERG. Causative genes include: *BEST1, C1QTNF5, EFEMP1, ELOVL4, FSCN2, GUCA1B, HMCN1, IMPG1, PROM1, PRPH2, RP1L1, TIMP3, ABCA4, CFH, IMPG1, RPGR*

Vitreoretinopathy: This includes individuals with familial exudative vitreoretin-opathy, retinal detachment (or traction), optically empty vitreous, fibrillary condensation, PHPV and neovascularization. Causative genes include: *COL11A1*, *COL2A1, COL9A1, FZD4, KCNJ13, LRP5, NDP, TSPAN12, VCAN*

Bardet–Biedl Syndrome: This includes individuals with retinal dystrophies, postaxial polydactyly, truncal obesity, learning disabilities, genitourinary abnormalities. Causative genes include: *ARL6, BBIP1, BBS1, BBS2, BBS4, BBS5, BBS7, BBS9, BBS10, BBS12, CEP290, IFT27, INPP5E, KCNJ13, LZTFL1, MKKS, MKS1, NPHP1, SDCCAG8, TRIM32, TTC8*

5. Ocular Tumors (Refer to Section 8 for more details)

1. Retinoblastoma

   a. This is the most common primary ocular malignancy in children before age five
   b. Gene has been identified as *RB1*. This tumor suppressor gene is recessive but there is a high rate of spontaneous mutation of this gene. Thus, both patients with and without germline RB1 mutation can develop retinoblastoma if both copies of the gene have become mutated
   c. The mutation may be sporadic (only within the tumor) or germline
   d. Current genetic testing can detect >85% of germ-line mutations. It is useful for screening at-risk family members who will undergo examination under anesthesia till age six, unless ruled out with genetic testing

      i. A patient with familial retinoblastoma has 100% chance of a germ-line mutation
      ii. If a patient with unilateral retinoblastoma has no family history of retinoblastoma, there is 15% chance the patient may have a germ-line mutation that may be detected by genetic testing

   e. It is important to identify patients with germ-line mutations since they are at risk for secondary tumors
   f. Genetic testing is done on the tumor and/or peripheral white blood cells
   g. The types of genetic testing for retinoblastoma include the following

      i. Sequence analysis of *RB1* gene
      ii. Comparative Genomic Hybridization array to detect deletions and duplications in *RB1*

        iii. Allele-specific Polymerase Chain Reaction (AS–PCR) for recurrent RB1 mutations

        iv. Testing for methylation of the *RB1* Promoter

  h. Among individuals that are negative for *RB1* gene testing, MYCN gene testing should be considered since mutation in this gene has been found in a smaller group of retinoblastoma patients

     (i) Quantitative multiplex PCR is carried out to identify *MYCN* copy number change in any tumor sample that does not have an *RB1* mutation

     (ii) Amplification of the MYCN oncogene has been detected in a new subset of retinoblastoma with early age of presentation and characterized by a distinct histology and no *RB1* mutations

2. Retinal angioma or hemangioblastoma

  a. This may present as an an isolated tumor in the retina or associated with Von Hippel–Lindau (VHL), a systemic disease

  b. Patients with VHL require regular systemic evaluation since systemic associated conditions can be life-threatening

  c. The genetic test for VHL gene mutation can diagnose Von Hippel–Lindau in 90 to 100% of cases of VHL, an autosomal dominant condition

  d. Genetic testing is useful to rule out systemic disease in patients without family history who present with a retinal angioma and for screening family members who are at risk of inheriting the disease

3. Uveal Melanoma

  a. Less than 2% of uveal melanoma cases could be ascribed to germ-line mutations in BRCA2, p16/p14, or p15

  b. Genetic profile and chromosomal abnormality of the tumor has been associated with prognosis (i.e. relative risk of metastatic disease)

  c. The genetic testing is used by some clinicians for determining frequency of screening for metastatic disease. For example, uveal melanoma demonstrating complete monosomy 3 has substantially poorer prognosis at 3 years than those with partial monosomy 3 or disomy 3. Similarly, choroidal melanoma with Class 2 genetic profile has 80 to 90% risk of metastasis

  d. Genetic analysis of the tumor prior to radiation or enucleation is recommended if patients are considering participating in adjuvant therapy clinical trials

Points to Remember about Genetic Testing

1. Genetic counseling prior to genetic testing is highly recommended
2. Many inherited diseases may not have a gene identified as yet
3. Without functional studies, many rare missense changes are reported as variants of unknown significance and may be confusing to patients
4. Next generation sequencing panels and microarrays have the potential of identifying changes in genes that can cause systemic conditions. Patients and families should be appropriately counseled about these incidental findings
5. Genetic findings in an individual have implications for the entire family
6. Genetic testing provides more accurate diagnosis for families but clinical trials and treatments are not yet available for the vast majority of individuals at this time. Gene therapy is available for only *RPE65* gene associated Leber congenital amaurosis, a rare condition that constitutes only a very small fraction of inherited retinal diseases that afflict patients
7. Do not forget to offer supportive visual management including referral for vision aids to improve patient's quality of life and referral to support groups

References

1. Retina Issue: The Proceedings of the First International Symposium on Translational Clinical Research for Inherited and Orphan Retinal Diseases: Sponsored by the National Neurovision Research Institute Inc. 2005;25(8).
2. Shankar SP. Hereditary Retinal and Choroidal Dystrophies. Emery and Rimoin's Principles and Practice of Medical Genetics, 6th edn., Elsevier Science (2013), Chapter 138, pp. 3888–3905.
3. Retrieved from
    OMIM.org.
    https://sph.uth.edu/Retnet/home.htm.
    https://www.genetests.org/.
    www.nei.nih.gov/resources/eyegene.asp.
    http://www.aao.org/publications/eyenet/201206/comprehensive.cfm.
4. Dollfus H, Massin P, Taupin P, *et al.* Retinal hemangioblastoma in von Hippel–Lindau disease: A clinical and molecular study. *Invest Ophthalmol Vis Sci* 2002;43(9): 3067–3074.
5. National Cancer Institute: Genetic Testing for Hereditary Cancer Syndromes. http://www.cancer.gov/cancertopics/factsheet/Risk/genetic-testing.
6. Hearle N, Damato BE, Humphreys J, Wixey J, Green, H, Stone J, Easton, DF, Houlston RS. Contribution of germline mutations in BRCA2, p16(INK4A), p14(ARF) and p15 to uveal melanoma. *Invest. Ophthal Vis Sci* 2003;44:458–462.
7. Shields CL(1), Ganguly A, Bianciotto CG, Turaka K, Tavallali A, Shields JA. Prognosis of uveal melanoma in 500 cases using genetic testing of fine-needle aspiration biopsy specimens. *Ophthalmol* 2011;118(2):396–401.

SECTION 2:
ACQUIRED MACULAR
DISORDERS

Chapter 4: Age-related Macular Degeneration

Gary Yau, David R.P. Almeida, Eric K. Chin and Susanna S. Park

1. Epidemiology of Age-related Macular Degeneration (AMD)

a. Leading cause of blindness in developed world
b. Accounts for >50% of blindness in U.S.
c. Prevalence by race in U.S.

- o 110 fold higher in white population compared to African-American

2. Initial Evaluation: Pertinent Details

- History
    - o Definite risk factors
        - Age: >50 years of age by definition
            - □ Incidence and severity of AMD increases with age
        - White race
        - Tobacco smoking
        - Family history of AMD
        - Sedentary lifestyle
        - Obesity
        - Cardiovascular disease (hypertension, hyperlipidemia)

o Symptoms

  ■ Often asymptomatic in early stage of AMD
  ■ Central visual disturbance, scotoma, metamorphopsia
  ■ Slowly progressive in dry AMD

    □ Acute worsening in wet AMD

o Eye Examination

  ■ Visual Acuity (ETDRS preferred over Snellen)
  ■ Fundus examination to classify stage of AMD:

    □ Early AMD

      — Few medium drusen ($\geq$63 μm to <125 μm)

    □ Intermediate AMD

      — Presence of pigmentary changes or large drusen ($\geq$125 μm)

    □ Late AMD

      — Neovascularization or geographic atrophy (GA)

    □ Subtypes of note

      — Drusenoid pigment epithelial detachment have high risk of conversion to late AMD (42% by 5 years) and should be followed closely

    □ Rare complications or presentations of neovascular AMD (NV-AMD)

      — Vitreous hemorrhage
      — Retinal pigment epithelial tears
      — Massive sub retinal hemorrhage

3. Major Differential Diagnosis of NV-AMD

• Polypoidal Choroidal Vasculopathy (PCV)

  o More common in non-Caucasians
  o Commonly misdiagnosed as NV-AMD
  o Characteristic recurrent serous, hemorrhagic and serosangenous pigment epithelial detachments
  o Indocyanine green (ICG) is used to confirm diagnosis (see below)

• (CSCR)

  o Atypical, chronic presentation in elderly patients may make diagnosis more challenging and difficult to differentiate from AMD

o Fluorescein angiography may show extensive areas of pigment alteration characteristic for this chronic phase of this condition
o Absence of drusen, supports this diagnosis

- Other etiologies of choroidal neovascular membrane (CNVM)

  o Trauma (choroidal rupture)
  o Myopia
  o Presumed ocular histoplasmosis (POHS)
  o Angioid Streaks

  ▪ Pseudoxanthoma Elasticum, Ehler-Danlos, Paget's Disease, Sickle Cell and other hemoglobinopathies, Idiopathic (PEPSI)

  o White Dot Syndromes

  ▪ Serpiginous, multifocal choroiditis, punctate inner choroiditis

  o Best's Disease
  o Idiopathic

4. Diagnostic Testing

- Non-exudative/dry AMD:

  o Clinical examination is adequate unless there is concern for conversion to NV-AMD

- Fluorescein angiography (FA)

  o The gold standard for diagnosing new NV-AMD
  o Types of neovascularization based on FA leakage has prognostic implications (Figures 1 and 2):

  1. Occult choroidal neovascularization

     a. Late leakage only
     b. Type 1 or sub-retinal pigment epithelial location usually

  2. Classic choroidal neovascularization

     a. Early well-defined area of hyperfluorescence with late leakage
     b. Type 2 or sub-retinal location usually

  3. Retinal angiomatous proliferation (RAP)

     a. Occult late leakage on FA with associated retinal hemorrhage
     b. Accounts for 20% of NV-AMD

    c. May have neovascularization that extends to sub retinal and sub-retinal pigment epithelial

○ Type of NV-AMD based on location has implications on treatment options:

    1. Subfoveal: neovascularization involves the fovea
    2. Juxtfoveal: neovascularization spares the fovea but located within 200 μm.
    3. Extrafoveal: neovascularization is beyond 200 μm from the fovea

- Optical Coherence Tomography (OCT)

  ○ Useful to screen for intra retinal or sub-retinal fluid in dry AMD eyes with new vision loss to rule out conversion to NV-AMD

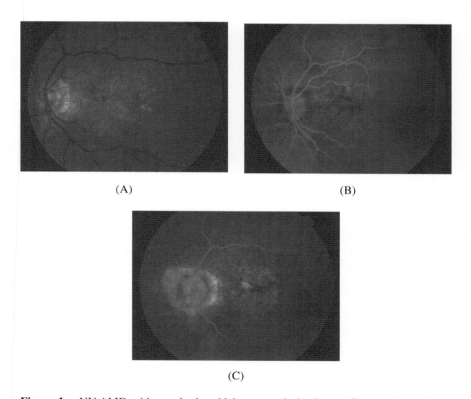

(A)   (B)

(C)

Figure 1. NV-AMD with occult choroidal neovascularization on fluorescein angiography. (A) Red-free photograph of the left macula shows some soft drusen and new blot retinal hemorrhages in this elderly patient with new visual complaints. (B) Early transit fluorescein angiogram of the left macula shows blockage from the macular hemorrhage. (C) Late transit fluorescein angiogram shows diffuse leakage around the hemorrhage.

o Useful to follow treatment response in eyes already diagnosed with NV-AMD

1. Quantitative features: central macular thickness (CMT)
2. Qualitative features: presence or absence of intra retinal fluid, retinal cystoid abnormalities, sub-retinal fluid, sub-RPE fluid

o Spectral-domain OCT has superior resolution compared to Time-domain OCT, and is capable of detecting more subtle qualitative intra retinal abnormalities, but the clinical significance of these findings are yet to be determined in AMD management

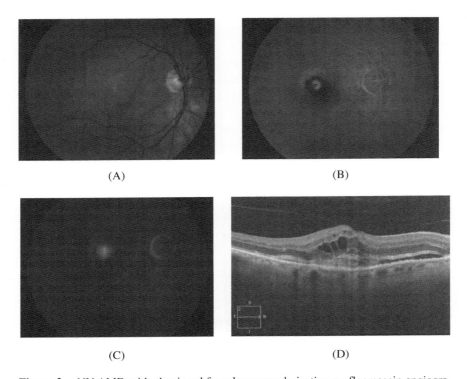

(A)   (B)

(C)   (D)

Figure 2. NV-AMD with classic subfoveal neovascularization on fluorescein angiography. (A) Red-free photography shows a small subfoveal lesion in this elderly woman with new visual loss in the right eye. (B) Early transit fluorescein angiogram shows a focal subfoveal area of early hyperfluorescence with well-defined borders and a rim of hypofluorescence. (C) Late transit angiogram shows diffuse subfoveal leakage consistent with a subfoveal neovascular membrane. (D) SD-OCT images shows a new hyperreflective sub retinal (type 2) lesion with mild macular edema and sub macular fluid.

- o Can be used in aiding diagnosis of RAP

    1. Intra retinal exudation: hyper-reflective deposits
    2. Intra retinal fluid

- Indocyanine Green Angiography (ICG)

    - o Can be used to help visualize sub retinal neovascularization associated with macular hemorrhage
    - o Can be used to differentiate from PCV

5. Management of Non-exudative (dry) AMD

- Amsler grid monitoring
- Smoking cessation
- Regular exercise and weight control
- Control and monitor blood pressure and lipid
- Diet rich in fresh fruits, green leafy vegetables and fish
- Minimize intake of processed food and fatty food
- Eye examination at least annually
- Intermediate or late AMD in at least one eye:

    - o Daily oral supplementation with antioxidant vitamins and minerals (AREDS formula)
    - o 500 mg vitamin C, 400 IU of vitamin E, 80 mg zinc oxide and 2 mg copper (cupric oxide)
    - o 10 mg lutein and 2 mg zeaxanthin is recommended as substitute for beta-carotene based on AREDS2 findings

- Late AMD with irreversible vision loss

    - o Low vision evaluation

6. Management of Exudative AMD (NV-AMD)

- Intravitreal anti-vascular endothelial growth factor (VEGF) therapy

    - o Indication: subfoveal or juxtafoveal NV-AMD if VA better than CF

        - FDA approved therapies:

            - □ Ranibizumab (0.5 mg) up to every 4 weeks
            - □ Aflibercept (2 mg) every 4 weeks for the first 3 months than every 8 weeks

- ■ Off-label therapies:

  - □ Bevacizumab (1.25 mg) as needed
  - □ Least expensive
  - □ Concerns about systemic side-effects but none noted in comparative clinical trials

  - o CATT and IVAN studies compared Bevacizumab and Ranibizumab and showed no difference in visual outcome after 2 years, but possible higher risk of geographic atrophy with ranibizumab although less fluid on OCT
  - o Relative contraindications to anti-VEGF therapy is recent stroke or uncontrolled hypertension
  - o A variety of treatment and re-treatment schemes exist:

    1. Monthly treatment is gold standard

       a. CATT and IVAN studies showed inferior visual outcome as needed dosing after 2 years

    2. Treat and extend is an alternative dosing being explored but no clinical data available on relative efficacy at current time

  - o Can be used alone or in combination with other treatments

- • Photodynamic therapy (PDT) with verteporfin

  - o Visual outcome is inferior to ranibizumab monotherapy but better than placebo for subfoveal classic NV-AMD (TAP Study)
  - o May be used with anti-VEGF therapy for resistant cases of subfoveal, classic NV-AMD, but visual outcome with combination therapy poorer than monotherapy in randomized clinical trials
  - o Combination with anti-VEGF therapy may be preferred over anti-VEGF monotherapy in eyes with PCV

- • Laser photocoagulation (Macular Photocoagulation Study)

  - o Indication: extrafoveal, classic CNVM
  - o May be used in conjunction with intravitreal anti-VEGF or corticosteroid to minimize risk of recurrence
  - o Advantage: more permanent therapy than anti-VEGF therapy

7. Prognosis is Based on Severity of AMD

- • Early AMD: 1/3rd will progress to intermediate AMD in 5 years

- Intermediate AMD: 1/2 will progress to late AMD by 5 years

  o AREDS supplementation reduces risk of developing advanced AMD by 25% at 5 years

- Late GA-AMD: 5–9 years to legal blindness
- Late NV-AMD: For those treated with anti-VEGF agents, 1/3rd have good visual outcomes (better than 20/70) and 1/3rd of poor visual outcomes by 7 years

References

1. Lim LS, Mitchell P, Seddon JM, *et al.* Age-related macular degeneration. *Lancet* 2012;379(9827):1728–1738.
2. Smith W, Assink J, Klein R, *et al.* Risk factors for age-related macular degeneration. Pooled findings from three continents. *Ophthalmol* 2001;108:697–704.
3. Congdon N, O'Colmain B, Klaver CC, *et al.* Eye Diseases Prevalence Research Group. Causes and prevalence of visual impairment among adults in the United States. *Arch Ophthalmol* 2004;122(4):477–485.
4. Friedman DS, Katz J, Bressler NM, *et al.* Racial differences in the prevalence of age-related macular degeneration: The Baltimore Eye Survey. *Ophthalmol* 1999;106: 1049–1055.
5. Ferris FL, Wilkinson CP, Bird A, *et al.* Clinical classification of age-related macular degeneration. *Ophthalmol* 2013;120:844–851.
6. Cukras C, Agron E, Klein ML, *et al.* Natural history of drusenoid pigment epithelial detachment in age-related macular degeneration: Age-related eye disease study Report No 28. *Ophthalmol* 2010;117(3):489–499.
7. Do DV, Gower EW, Cassard SD, *et al.* Detection of new-onset choroidal neovascularization using optical coherence tomography: The AMD DOC study. *Ophthalmol* 2012;119:771–778.
8. Khurana RN, Dupas B, Bressler NM. Agreement of time-domain and spectral-domain optical coherence tomography with fluorescein leakage from choroidal neovascularization. *Ophthalmol* 2010;117(7):1376–1380.
9. Stanga PE, Li JL, Hamilton P. Indocyanine green angiography in chorioretinal diseases: An evidence-based update. *Ophthalmol* 2003;110(1):15–21.
10. Yannuzzi LA. Indocyanine green angiography. A perspective on use in the clinical setting. *Am J Ophthalmol* 2011;151:745–751.
11. The age-related eye disease study 2 (AREDS2) research group. Lutein + zeaxanthin and omega-3 fatty acids for age-related macular degeneration. The age-related eye disease study 2 (AREDS2) randomized clinical trial. *JAMA* 2013;209(10):2005–2015.
12. CATT. Ranibizumab and bevacizumab for treatment of neovascular age-related macular degeneration. Two-year results. *Ophthalmol* 2012;119:1388–1398.
13. Heier JS, Brown DM, Chong V, *et al.* Intravitreal aflibercept (VEGF Trap-eye) in wet age-related macular degeneration. *Ophthalmol* 2012;119:2537–2548.
14. Bressler NM. Photodynamic therapy of subfoveal choroidal neovascularization in age-related macular degeneration with verteporfin: Two-year results of 2 randomized clinical trials-tap report 2. *Arch Ophthalmol* 2001;119:198–207.
15. Japanese age-related macular degeneration trial (JAT) study group. Japanese age-related macular degeneration trial: One-year results of photodynamic therapy with verteporfin in Japanese patients with subfoveal choroidal neovascularization secondary to age-related macular degeneration. *Am J Ophthalmol* 2003;136(6):1049–1061.

16. Macular Photocoagulation Study Group. Argon laser photocoagulation for neovascular maculopathy. Three-year results from randomized clinical trials. *Arch Ophthalmol* 1986;104:694–701.

17. Hooper P, Jutai JW, Strong G, *et al.* Age-related macular degeneration and low-vision rehabilitation: A systematic review. *Can J Ophthalmol* 2008;43(2):180–187.

18. Rasmussen A, Bloch SB, Fuchs J, *et al.* A 4-year longitudinal study of 555 patients treated with ranibizumab for neovascular age-related macular degeneration. *Ophthalmol* 2013;S0161–6420.

19. The Age-Related Eye Disease Study Research Group. A randomized, placebo-controlled, clinical trial of high-dose supplementation with vitamins C and E, beta carotene, and zinc for age-related macular degeneration and vision loss: AREDS report no. 8. *Arch Ophthalmol* 2001;119:1417–1436.

20. Grunwald JE, Pistelli M, Ying G, *et al.* For the Comparison of Age-related Macular Degeneration Treatment Trials Research Group. Growth of geographic atrophy in the Comparison of Age-related Macular Degeneration Treatment Trials. *Ophthalmol* 2014.

Chapter 5: Central Serous Chorioretinopathy

Gary Yau, David R.P. Almeida, Eric K. Chin and Susanna S. Park

1. Epidemiology: Central Serous Chorioretinopathy (CSCR)

- Mean age: 41–45 years
- Annual incidence of 10/100 000 in men
- Men to Women ratio: 6:1

2. Initial Evaluation: Pertinent History

Identify any known associations

- Exogenous corticosteroid use

  o May be primary use or even unintentional secondary exposure

- Elevated endogenous corticosteroid levels

  o Cushing's syndrome, Pregnancy, Type A personality

- Recent psychosocial stressors
- Sleep apnea

3. Presenting Signs and Symptoms

- Central distortion (metamorphopsia)
- Acquired hypermetropia
- Other: micropsia, reduced contrast sensitivity, acquired dyschromatopsia
- Visual Acuity: 20/20 to 20/200

4. Clinical Findings

Acute phase

- Macular serous neurosensory detachment
- Often associated with pigment epithelial detachments and associated retinal pigment epithelium (RPE) changes which may be more visible on fluorescein angiography
- Small subset may have fibrous exudate
- Can be multifocal or bifocal
- Absence of macular hemorrhage

Chronic phase

- Defined as serous retinal detachment (SRD) that has not resolved by 3 months
- Shallow SRD with diffuse retinal pigment epitheliopathy, geographic atrophy, chronic intra retinal cystic changes
- May have "bullous" SRD gravitating inferiorly leaving tracts of sub retinal fluid and pigment changes

5. Differential Diagnosis for Intra Retinal or Sub Retinal Macular Fluid

- Polypoidal choroidal vasculopathy (PCV)
- NV-AMD
- Optic nerve pit maculopathy
- Other causes: inflammatory, infectious, autoimmune, vascular and intra ocular tumors

6. Diagnostic Testing (Figure 1)

Optical Coherence Tomography (OCT)

- Useful for diagnosing neurosensory detachment and possible associated retinal pigment epithelial detachments
- Intra retinal fluid and cystic changes may be noted in chronic phase of CSCR
- Increased choroid thickness measurements has been reported via enhanced depth imaging OCT

Fluorescein Angiography

- Useful for diagnosis and to differentiate from other causes of macular fluid
- Needed to establish targets (focal leaks) for laser therapy

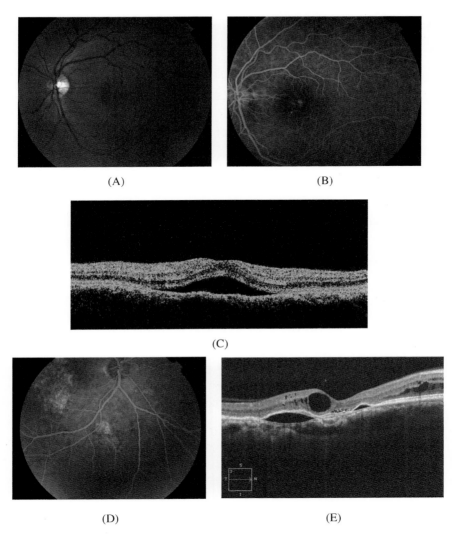

Figure 1. Retinal imaging of acute versus chronic CSCR. (A) A red-free fundus photo of a patient with recent vision loss from CSCR showing mild elevation of the central macula from sub-retinal fluid. (B) Mid transit fluorescein angiogram of this patient with recent vision loss shows multifocal leakage near the fovea. (C) OCT imaging shows sub-retinal fluid without intra retinal fluid is typically seen in eyes with this more acute condition. (D) Mid phase fluorescein angiogram of this elderly man with chronic intra retinal, sub-retinal fluid and pigment epithelial detachment simulating active sub-retinal neovascularization shows multiple diffuse areas of mottled staining extending inferiorly outside the macula without clear pinpoint leakage, consistent with chronic CSCR. (E) Spectral-domain OCT shows the residual intra retinal and sub-retinal fluid which was resistant to antiVEGF therapy but resolved fully with oral finesteride.

Acute CSCR

- Features

  o Focal leakage associated with SRD

    ▪ Most common: expansile dot — commonly multifocal
    ▪ Smokestack
    ▪ Can be used to direct targets for focal argon therapy

  o Pigment epithelial detachment noted in 5%

Chronic CSCR

- Features of retinal pigment epitheliopathy
- Associated vascular changes: capillary dropout, telangiectasia may be also seen

Indocyanine Green Angiography

- May be considered in chronic or atypical cases
- Typical sequence

  1. Early hypofluorescence (localized delay in arterial filing)
  2. Dilatation of choroidal vessels
  3. Mid-phase hyperfluorescence
  4. Late phase washout

- May show areas of choroidal leakage not seen by FA that can be used as targets for laser for PDT

7. Management

- Minimize any identified associated risk factors if possible
- Lifestyle changes for better stress management may be indicated

Acute; first episode

- Observe for 3 months and consider treatment if condition persists
- Indications for earlier treatment

  o Monocular
  o Recurrent disease

- Occupational needs for quicker visual recovery
- Previous disease in fellow eye requiring therapy

If chronic, consider the following treatment options

1. Focal argon photocoagulation

   a. Need recent (within 1 week) fluorescein angiography to guide treatment

      - Focal extrafoveal leaks are targeted
      - RPE defects with associated leakage
      - Argon laser

        1. Spot size: 100–200 μm
        2. Duration: 100 msec
        3. Power (low): 100–200 mW
        4. Target appearance: slight greying of retina
        5. 3 to 5 spots directly at site of leakage

   b. Shown to hasten recovery, should see resolution of leakage in 2 weeks, however, final visual outcome similar to natural history
   c. Major complications

      - 10% risk of choroidal neovascular membrane
      - Permanent scotomas

2. Photodynamic therapy (PDT) with verteporfin

   a. Advantages over focal laser photocoagulation

      - Can treat eyes without focal leakage on angiography
      - Less risk of choroidal neovascularization or permanent scotoma

   b. Variable settings have been used but reduced dose and lower fluence appear to have similar efficacy to full fluence with less risk of side effects
   c. IV Verteporfin Dose

      - Standard-dose (6.0 mg/m^2 of body surface area)
      - **Half-dose** (3.0 mg/m^2 of body surface area)
      - Infuse over 10 minutes, then wait 5 minutes for PDT

   d. Laser parameters, using diode laser wavelength 689 nm:

      - Standard-fluence: 50 mJ/cm^2, 600 mW, over 83 seconds
      - **Half-fluence**: 25–35 mJ/cm^2, 600 mW, 83 seconds
      - Spot size: diameter large enough to cover entire lesion

e. Major complications:

- Verteporfin-related skin burn: patient should avoid direct sun exposure or bright indoor lights for 5 days after treatment
- Back pain during verteporfin infusion: minimized with adequate hydration prior to treatment

8. Follow-up and Monitoring

- If active, assess for resolution of SRD in 6 weeks to 3 months using serial OCT
- If inactive, asses every 3 months to 1 year with OCT or sooner as needed
- Amsler grid home monitoring

9. Prognosis

- Most acute CSCR will resolve by 3 months without significant visual loss
- 31% of eyes will have recurrence, with a median time frame of 1.3 years (range 0.4–18.2) from first episode
- Worse prognosis correlated with

  o Older age at presentation (>50)
  o Worse visual acuity at presentation
  o Duration of chronicity

- Focal laser and PDT hasten recovery, but there is a lack of study showing benefit of treatment in terms of final visual outcome or reduction in rate of recurrence compared to observation alone

References

1. Lieu G, Quin G, Gillies M, *et al.* Central serous chorioretinopathy: A review of epidemiology and pathophysiology. *Clin Experimental Ophthalmol* 2013;41:201–214.
2. Quin G, Lieu G, Ho I, *et al.* Diagnosis and interventions for central serous chorioretinopathy: Review and update. *Clin Experimental Ophthalmol* 2013;41:187–200.
3. Nicholson B, Noble J, Forooghian F, *et al.* Central serous chorioretinopathy: Update on pathophysiology and treatment. *Surv Ophthalmol* 2013;58(2):103–126.
4. Kitzmann AS, Pulido JS, Diehl NN, *et al.* The incidence of central serous chorioretinopathy in Olmsted County, Minnesota, 1980–2002. *Ophthalmol* 2008;115:169–173.
5. Mudvari SS, Goff MJ, Fu AD, *et al.* The natural history of pigment epithelial detachment associated with central serous chorioretinopathy. *Retina* 2007;27(9):1168–1173.
6. Schatz H, McDonald HR, Johnson RN, *et al.* Sub-retinal fibrosis in central serous chorioretinopathy. *Ophthalmol* 1995;102(7):1077–1088.
7. Spaide RF, Campeas L, Haas A *et al.* Central serous chorioretinopathy in younger and older adults. *Ophthalmol* 1996;103:2070–2079.
8. Lim JI, Glassman AR, Aiello LP, *et al.* Collaborative retrospective macula society study of photodynamic therapy for chronic central serous chorioretinopathy. *Ophthalmol* 2014;121(5):1073–1078.
9. Imamura Y, Fujiwara T, Margolis R, *et al.* Enhanced depth imaging optical coherence tomography of the choroid in central serous chorioretinopathy. *Retina* 2011;29:1469–1473.
10. Liu DT, Fok AC, Chan W, *et al.* Central serous chorioretinopathy. In Retina textbook, SJ Ryan, 5th edn, Mosby (Maryland, U.S.) 2013;72:1296.
11. Thinda S, Lam K, Park SS. Unintentional Secondary Exogenous Corticosteroid Exposure and Central Serous Chorioretinopathy. *Eye.*

Chapter 6: Epiretinal Membrane

Gary Yau, David R.P. Almeida, Eric K. Chin
and Susanna S. Park

1. Epidemiology of Epiretinal Membrane (ERM)

- Prevalence

  o 2% in <60 years old
  o 12% in >70 years old

- 5-year cumulative incidence

  o 1.5–3.8%

- Bilateral in up to 30%
- Idiopathic: most common etiology

2. Pertinent Signs and Symptoms

- Gradual loss of visual acuity: 20/20 to counting fingers

  o Central distortion: metamorphopsia, monocular diplopia

- Clinical findings:

  o Cellophane maculopathy: sheen of translucent membrane with no wrinkling of inner macula
  o Partial or Full thickness folding of macular retina, may induce distortion of superficial retinal vessels
  o Can have underlying microvascular retinal changes from traction on the retinal vessels

o Lamellar or pseudohole, with negative Watze-Allen sign (contrary to full-thickness macular hole)
o Usually associated with a posterior vitreous detachment

3. Major Non-idiopathic Causes

- Iatrogenic

  o Intraocular surgery: cataract surgery, retinal surgery, silicone oil
  o Intraocular laser photocoagulation or cryotherapy

- Inflammatory retinal or choroidal disease
- Vascular occlusive disease

  o Diabetic retinopathy, retinal vein occlusion, idiopathic macular telangiectasia, retinal arteriolar macro-aneurysms, sickle cell retinopathy

- Trauma
- Retinal detachment
- Other: tumor, retinal dystrophies, retinal angiomas, hamartomas, retinitis pigmentosa

4. Diagnostic Testing

Optical Coherence Tomography (OCT)

- ERM is seen as hyper-reflective layer on inner retinal surface with associated changes to underlying retina (Figure 1)
- Concurrent changes in the macula may be seen

  o vitremacular traction (VMT)
  o cystoid macular edema (CME)
  o macular schisis
  o macular surface wrinkling

- Visual acuity loss has been correlated best with increased foveal thickness or disruption on OCT and necessarily with macular thickening

Fluorescein angiography

- Can differentiate non-idiopathic causes of ERM and better characterize vascular components that may be contributing to macular thickening

5. Management

- Indications for surgery vary, but generally dictated by visual function
  - o Typically visual acuity of 20/60 or worse. More recent onset are considered best candidates if no other cause of vision loss
- Poor presentation visual acuity and long duration of symptoms are associated with poorer visual outcomes after surgery
- Surgery for ERM
  - o Pars plana subtotal or total vitrectomy
    - ▪ Subtotal vitrectomy theoretically may decrease risk of cataract and peripheral retinal tears
  - o Membrane removal of ERM and/or internal limiting membrane (ILM)
    - ▪ Straining allows improved visualization of membrane to be removed
    - ▪ Intravitreal triamcinolone (usually diluted 1:10 with balanced salt solution (BSS))
      - □ Allows improved visualization of ERM but not ILM
      - □ May improve rate of resolution of macular edema after surgery

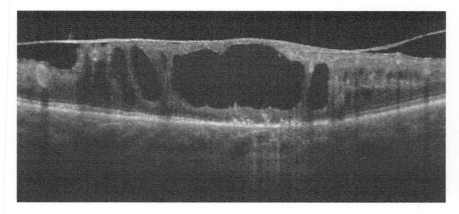

Figure 1. Spectral-domain OCT imaging of macular ERM. Note the diffuse hyperreflective line representing ERM which is adherent to the underlying thickened macula centrally and causing traction in this patient with longstanding central retinal vein occlusion and concurrent associated chronic macular edema.

      □ Intravitreal Brilliant Blue G (BBG) (0.2 mL of 0.25 mg/mL) or Indocyanine Green (use minimum concentration: 0.125%), used to negatively stain ILM around ERM

      □ Need prompt wash-out to minimize retinal toxicity

      □ Concurrent ILM removal has been advocated for more complete ERM removal and to minimize rate of recurrent ERM

      □ Re-staining may be needed if residual ERM or ILM is suspected

      □ Can consider double staining and "double peeling"

    ■ Check periphery 360 degrees for retinal tears

- Complications of vitrectomy:

    o Cataract progression, residual post-operative macular edema, recurrent ERM recurrence, macular hole, retinal detachment, endophthalmitis

6. Follow-up and Monitoring

If patient is asymptomatic or visual acuity is 20/40 or better

- Amsler grid monitoring for changes in metamorphopsia
- Serial appointments to assess visual acuity and morphologic changes in OCT
- Every 3 to 12 months

If following vitrectomy:

- Routine postoperative visits
- Visual acuity and OCT improvement may not be noted in the first 3 months and improvements may continue for a couple of years after surgery

7. Prognosis for ERM

- Natural history of ERM: stable or slow progression over years
- Visual outcome post-ERM vitrectomy surgery

    o Improvement of 2 or more lines in 65%

      ■ Anatomic recurrence in 10%

      ■ Re-operation required in 3%

References

1. Mitchell P, Smith W, Chey T, *et al*. Prevalence and associations of epiretinal membranes. The Blue Mountains Eye Study, Australia. *Ophthalmol* 1997;104:1033–1040.
2. Fraser-Bell S, Guzowski M, Rochtchina E, *et al*. Five-year cumulative incidence and progression of epiretinal membranes: The Blue Mountains Eye Study. *Ophthalmol* 2003;110:34–40.
3. Goldberg RA, Waheed NK and Duker JS. Optical coherence tomography in the preoperative and postoperative management of macular hole and epiretinal membrane. *Br J Ophthalmol* 2014;98:ii20–23.
4. Wickham L and Gregor Z. Epiretinal membranes. In Retina textbook, SJ Ryan, 5th edn., Mosby (Maryland, US) 2013;116:1959.
5. Carpentier C, Zanolli M, Wu L, *et al*. Residual internal limiting membrane after epiretinal membrane peeling: Results of the Pan-American Collaborative Retina Study Group. *Retina* 2013;33(10):2026–2031.
6. Park DW, Dugel PU, Garda J, *et al*. Macular pucker removal with and without internal limiting membrane peeling: Pilot study. *Ophthalmol* 2003;110:62–64.
7. Shimada H, Nakashuzuka H, Hattori T, *et al*. Double staining with brilliant blue G and double peeling for epiretinal membranes. *Ophthalmol* 2009;116(7):1370–1376.
8. Appiah AP, Hirose T, Kado M: A review of 324 cases of idiopathic premacular gliosis. *Am J Ophthalmol* 1988;106:533–535.
9. Sandali O, El Sanharawi M, Basli E, *et al*. Epiretinal membrane recurrence: Incidence, characteristics, evolution, and preventive and risk factors. *Retina* 2013;33(10):2032–2038.
10. Dawson SR, Shunmugam M, Williamson TH. Visual acuity outcomes following surgery for idiopathic epiretinal membrane: An analysis of data from 2001 to 2011. *Eye* 2014;28(2):219–224.
11. Pilli S, Lim P, Zawadzki RJ, *et al*. Fourier-domain optical coherence tomography of eyes with epiretinal membrane: Correlation between morphologic changes and visual function. *Eye* 2011;25:775–783.

Chapter 7: Macular Holes

**Gary Yau, David R.P. Almeida, Eric K. Chin
and Susanna S. Park**

1. Epidemiology of Full-thickness Macular Hole (FTMH)

- Age: typically >65 years
- Incidence 8 per 100,000 per year
- 2/3rd females
- 80% unilateral
- Etiology:

  - Idiopathic: 90%
  - Traumatic: 10%
  - Other (rare): myopia, VMT

2. Signs and Symptoms

- Semi-acute progressive loss of central vision.
- Presenting visual acuity: 20/20 to counting fingers

  - May be asymptomatic at early stage
  - Pincushion metamorphosia
  - Central scotoma

- Funduscopic findings vary with stage of Macular Hole

Gass classification of Macular Hole:

  - Stage 1a: yellow dot
  - Stage 1b: yellow ring
  - Stage 2: eccentric full-thickness macular hole (FTMH) <400 μm

    o   Stage 3: central FTMH >400 μm
    o   Stage 4: FTMH with posterior vitreous detachment (PVD)

Assess fellow-eye for prognostic reasons:

   Normal macula without PVD: 5-year incidence of FTMH is 15.6%
   Presence of PVD: <2 % risk of FTMH

3. Major Differential Diagnosis

Can differentiate based on funduscopy and OCT

a. Lamellar holes
b. Pseudohole with Epiretinal Membrane
c. Foveal cyst

4. Diagnostic Testing

OCT

- Can be used to diagnose anatomically, the stage of the macular hole (Figure 1)
- Can determine hole size

    o   Small ($\leq$250 μm)
    o   Medium (>250 to $\leq$400 μm)
    o   Large (>400 μm)

- Can detect associated Vitreo Macular Traction (VMT) or epiretinal membrane

Fluorescein Angiography

- Usually not necessary for diagnosis
- Can help rule out non-idiopathic causes of macular hole or other concurrent maculopathy or retinal vasculopathy which may be visually significant

5. Management of Macular Hole

a. Vitrectomy Surgery has been shown to close macular hole and improve vision in >90% of cases

   i. Considerations for case selection and timing of surgery:

- Duration of macular hole
- Ideally <6 months

- Worse visual prognosis if duration >2 years
- Stage of hole
- Surgery not indicated for Stage 1 hole since 50% chance for spontaneous recovery
- Stage 2 to 4 holes benefit from surgery: better prognosis for visual outcome and hole closure with smaller and earlier stage hole with shorter duration
- Ability to perform postoperative face down positioning

  Postoperative positioning improves success of surgery

o If patient is unable and hole is small with VMT, trial of intravitreal ocriplasmin can be considered (Jetrea) 0.125 mg
o Most effective for holes <250 μm, in absence of ERM

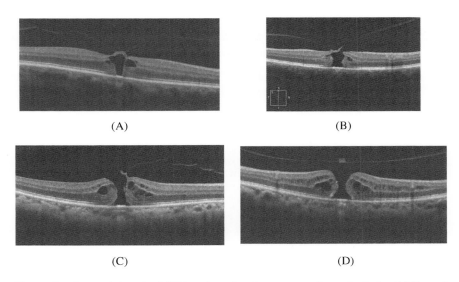

(A)   (B)

(C)   (D)

Figure 1. Spectral-domain OCT imaging of various stages of macular hole. (A) Stage 1 (impending) macular hole shows a foveal detachment from VMT with adjacent cystic changes in the central macula. (B) Stage 2 macular hole shows the eccentric small full-thickness retinal defect with associated VMT. (C) Stage 3 macular hole shows a larger full thickness macular defect with associated VMT. (D) Stage 4 macular hole shows a more centrally located full thickness macular defect with a pseudo-operculum contiguous with the posterior hyaloid face which is separated from the macula.

b. Vitrectomy surgical technique

- Pars Plana Vitrectomy (PPV) with separation of posterior vitreous cortex from retinal surface

  o Consider intravitreal triamcinolone acetonide for enhanced visualization of posterior hyaloid
  o If present, peel ERM
  o Consider peeling of inner limiting membrane (ILM) especially for Stage 3 to 4 holes

    ▪ Improves anatomic and functional outcomes.
    ▪ Caution: risk of retinal injury and toxicity
    ▪ Consider staining of ILM using indocyanine green (ICG) dye

      ▫ Varied reports on its advantages and potential toxicity
      ▫ Suggest concentration 0.25 to 0.5 mg/mL, in small volumes (<0.1 cc) in fluid filled eyes, short exposure times (<30 seconds), iso-osmolar solutions, and limit proximal or prolonged endo illumination of stained tissue

    ▪ Can substitute brilliant blue G (0.25 mg/mL) to be used in a similar fashion, but not yet FDA-approved in U.S.
    ▪ Trypan blue has been FDA-approved for this indication but weaker staining than ICG

- **Check periphery** for retinal tears with scleral depression

  o Predilection for inferior retinal breaks after separation of posterior vitreous detachment

- **Air-fluid exchange**, followed by gas exchange and Tamponade
- Gas Tamponade and Posturing

  o The type of gas and length of posturing has not been established Varying combinations have been suggested, with a trend towards shorter-acting and shorter face-down positioning
  o Most commonly used tamponade is SF_6 with 5–7 days of face down (prone) positioning
  o If face down positioning is not possible, recurrent macular hole, or need to travel to high altitude, consider silicone oil Tamponade

- Potential complications:

  o Cataract progression
  o Peripheral retinal breaks or detachment

o Peripheral visual field defects
o Re-opening of macular holes
o Endophthalmitis

6. Follow-up and Monitoring

- Serial appointments with OCT to monitor for improvement or possible progression

7. Prognosis after Vitrectomy for Macular Hole

- Hole closure can be seen on clinical examination within the first month.

  o Successful anatomic outcomes = 85–100%

- Mean postoperative visual acuity 20/40

  o Visual acuity may continue to improve during the first 2 years following surgery

References

1. Steel DHW, Lotery AJ. Idiopathic vitreomacular traction and macular hole: A comprehensive review of pathophysiology, diagnosis, and treatment. *Eye* 2013;27:S1–21.
2. Bainbridge J, Herbert E, Gregor Z. Macular holes. Vitreoretinal relationships and surgical approaches. *Eye* 2008;22:1301–1309.
3. McCannel CA, Ensminger JL, Diehl NN, *et al.* Population based incidence of macular holes. *Ophthalmol* 2009;116:1366–1369.
4. Ezra E, Wells JA, Gray RH, *et al.* Incidence of idiopathic full thickness macular holes in fellow eyes. A 5-year prospective natural history study. *Ophthalmol* 1998;105: 353–359.
5. Ezra E. Idiopathic full thickness macular hole: Natural history and pathogenesis. *Br J Ophthalmol* 2001;85:102–108.
6. Duker JS, Kaiser PK, Binder S, *et al.* The international vitreomacular traction study group classification of vitreomacular adhesion, traction, and macular hole. *Ophthalmol* 2013;120(12):2611–2619.
7. Benson WE, Cruickshanks KC, Fong DS, *et al.* Ophthalmic technology assessment. Surgical management of macular holes. A report by the American Academy of Ophthalmology. *Ophthalmol* 2001;108:1328–1335.
8. Stalmans P, Benz MS, Gandorfer A, *et al.* Enzymatic vitreolysis with ocriplasmin for vitreomacular traction and macular holes. *N Engl J Med* 2012;367(7):606–615.
9. Williams GA. Macular holes: The latest in current management. *Retina* 2006;26(6): S9–12.
10. Gaudric A, Tadayoni R. Macular hole. In Retina textbook, SJ Ryan, 5th edn, Mosby (Maryland, US) 2013;117:1969.
11. Cornish KS, Lois N, Scott NW *et al.* Vitrectomy with internal limiting membrane peeling versus non peeling for idiopathic full-thickness macular hole. *Ophthalmol* 2014;121:649–655.
12. Stanescu-Segall D, Jackson TL. Vital staining with indocyanine green: A review of the clinical and experimental studies relating to safety. *Eye* 2009;23(3):504–518.
13. Park SS, Marcus DM, Duker JS, *et al.* Posterior segment complications following vitreous surgery for macular hole. *Ophthalmol* 1995;102:775–781.
14. Solebo AL, Lange CA, Bunce C, *et al.* Face-down positioning or posturing after macular hole surgery. *Cochrane Database Syst Rev* 2011;12.
15. Jackson TL, Donachie PH, Sparrow JM, *et al.* United Kingdom National Ophthalmology database study of vitreoretinal surgery: Report 2, macular hole. *Ophthalmol* 2013;120(3):629–634.
16. Pilli S, Zawadzki RJ, Werner JS, *et al.* Visual outcome correlates with inner macular volume in eyes with surgically closed macular hole. *Retina* 2012;32:2085–2095.

Chapter 8:
Toxic Maculopathy/Retinopathy

Gary Yau, David R.P. Almeida, Eric K. Chin and Susanna S. Park

AMINOQUINOLINE (CHLOROQUINE AND HYDROXYCHLOROQUINE) TOXICITY

1. Epidemiology

- Incidence rare, but increases with daily dose, cumulative dose, and duration of treatment
- 350,000 patients in the U.S. are at risk and must undergo screening
- Using 2002 screening criteria:
  - o 1% incidence after 5–7 years of therapy, or cumulative dose of 1,000 g
- Using 2011 AAO screening criteria:
  - o 7.5% incidence after >5 years
  - o 2% incidence in the first 10 years with daily dose of 4–5 mg/kg
  - o 20% incidence after 20 years with daily dose of 4–5 mg/kg

2. Indications for Chloroquine or Hydroxychloroquine Use

- Rheumatoid arthritis (RA)
- Systemic lupus erythematosus (SLE)
- Sjogren's syndrome
- Photodermatitis
- Malaria prophylaxis
- Oncology
- Amebiasis

3. Risk Factors for Macular Toxicity

- Daily dose of drug

  - o Controversial whether it should be based on ideal weight, actual weight or serum levels of drug to minimize toxicity (2012 AAO guideline recommends ideal body weight)
  - o Chloroquine >3 mg/kg/day
  - o Hydroxychloroquine >6.5 mg/kg/day

    - ▪ *Note*: Most are prescribed 400 mg/day, which is acceptable for most patients, except those with short stature, generally less than 5'2" if calculating based on ideal body weight

- Cumulative dose (life time)

  - o Chloroquine >100 g
  - o Hydroxychloroquine >1,000 g

- Cumulative duration of treatment

  - o >5 years

- Concurrent macular disorder

  - o ABCA4 gene mutation may be linked with increased risk of toxicity

    - ▪ Concurrent use of other toxic medications i.e. tamoxifen

- Renal or liver disease
- Older age (>60)
- Obesity

4. Clinical Signs and Symptoms

- May be asymptomatic at early stages when the condition is more likely to be reversible
- Symptomatic at later stages:

  - o Metamorphopsia
  - o Central or paracentral scotoma
  - o Acquired dyschromatosia
  - o Loss of vision
  - o Photophobia
  - o Nyctalopia
  - o Other (secondary to corneal and lenticular effects): glareness, blurred vision

- Signs
  - o External: depigmentation of the lid or lashes
  - o Cornea: verticillata
    - ▪ More common with chloroquine
    - ▪ Reversible
  - o Lens: cataract
  - o Retina:
    - ▪ Early: mild perifoveal depigmentation of the RPE
    - ▪ Late: bull's eye maculopathy, concurrent cystoid macular edema possible (Figure 1)
    - ▪ Very late: diffuse retinal degeneration with pigment changes

5. Differential Diagnosis for Bull's Eye Maculopathy

- Age related Macular Degeneration (AMD)
- Chronic macular hole
- Cone dystrophy, cone-rod dystrophy
- Stargardt's disease
- Central areolar choroidal atrophy
- Benign concentric annular dystrophy
- Batton's disease

6. Clinical Examination and Diagnostic Testing

- Best corrected visual acuity and comprehensive dilated eye examination
- 2011 Screening guidelines from the AAO recommends combining one functional and one structural test at baseline and screening with follow-up visits
  - o Functional tests recommended:
    - ▪ Humphrey visual field 10–2
      - ☐ White stimulus recommended
      - ☐ Red stimulus less specific
    - ▪ Multifocal ERG
      - ☐ Most sensitive but least available

o Structural tests recommended:

- SD-OCT (spectral domain optical coherence tomography) (Figure 1)

  □ Perifoveal blurring, disruption or loss of the photoreceptor inner segment-outer segment (i.e. ellipsoid) line leading to "flying saucer sign" in more advanced stage

  □ Macular thickness map: thinning of the perifoveal ETDRS zones

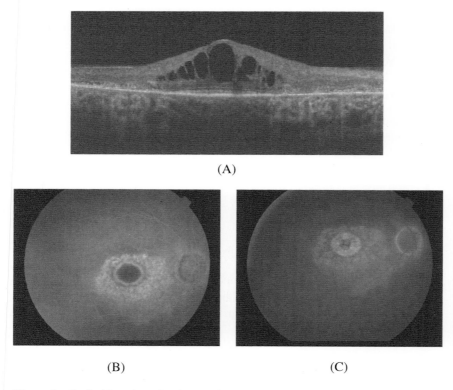

(A)

(B)   (C)

Figure 1. Retinal imaging of toxic maculopathy associated with chronic hydroxychloroquine use. (A) Spectral-domain OCT imaging showing the characteristic loss of the perifoveal photoreceptor inner segment-outer segment (ellipsoid) zone with foveal preservation. Concurrent cystoid macular edema is seen in this patient with visual acuity of 20/50. Clinical examination shows bull's eye maculopathy. (B) Mid transit fluorescein angiogram showing mottled hyperfluorescence in the bull's eye configuration. (C) Late transit fluorescein angiogram shows additional central petelloid hyperfluorescence from concurrent angiographic cystoid macular edema.

  □ May be more sensitive than perimetry or autofluoresence in some eyes
  □ Commonly used structural test since fast and readily available

- Autofluoresence

  □ New hyper- or hypo-fluorescence changes in the perifoveal zone may be significant

• Fundus photography and fluorescein angiography (Figure 1)

  o Not indicated for routine screening
  o Indicated only in more advanced cases to rule out other causes of bull's eye maculopathy

7. 2011 Screening Guidelines and Management

a. If normal baseline eye examination at time of initiation of drug

  • Follow-up screening recommendations in 5 years after starting chronic amino quinolone therapy, then annually thereafter
  • More frequent screening is recommended if any risk factors are present or any changes in drug dose occurs

b. If an abnormal baseline eye examination and/or diagnostic test is noted

  • Consult an internist or rheumatologist with regards to ideal medication regimen and consider changing medication if possible
  • If no change in medication is feasible, every 6 month screening and consider stopping medication if there are any signs of change

c. New abnormal screening examination after starting medication

  • Discuss with internist and consider cessation of drug and initiation of alternative therapy
  • Close follow-up every 3 days if drug is continued
  • Follow-up every 6–12 months for signs of reversal or worsening if the drug is stopped

8. Prognosis

• Toxic maculopathy or retinopathy can be reversible if diagnosed early and drug discontinued promptly
• Advanced toxic maculopathy is not reversible and likely progressive even after stopping the drug since it can take 3 to 6 months for the drug to completely clear from body upon cessation

- There are reports of delayed onset of toxic retinopathy up to 7 years after discontinuation of drug

PHENOTHIAZINE TOXICITY

1. Phenothiazine Subtypes

- **Thioridazine** — more common cause of toxicity
- **Chlorpromazine** — less common cause of retinal toxicity

  - Need very high doses for retinal toxicity

2. Indications for Phenothiazine Use

- Anti-psychotic therapy

3. Risk Factor for Retinal Toxicity

- High daily drug dose:

  - Thioridazine >800 mg/day
  - Chlorpromazine: >2,400 mg/day

4. Signs and Symptoms of Retinal Toxicity

- New visual complaints with onset, within weeks of drug to drug toxic daily doses

  - There are rare reports of delayed toxic reaction from cumulative dose
  - Complaints may vary from blurry vision, acquired dyschromatopsia, Nyctalopia

- Fundus changes suggestive of toxicity

  - Early: course, granular pigment stippling
  - Intermediate: patchy or nummular areas of RPE loss
  - Late: widespread areas of depigmentation with hyper pigmented plaques associated with vascular attenuation (and associated optic atrophy)

- Other associated findings with chlorpromazine: anterior stellate lens opacities

5. Diagnostic Testing

- Fluorescein angiography may be used to rule out other causes of visual loss or fundus pigment alteration

- OCT may be useful to detect disruption in photoreceptor layer
- ERG will help diagnose widespread photoreceptor abnormality

6. Management

- Cessation of medication is recommended at the earliest sign of toxicity after discussion with psychiatrist regarding alternative medical therapy

7. Prognosis and Follow-up

- Typical visual function improves after cessation. There is a low risk of gradual progressive loss of visual function after drug cessation
- Follow-up evaluation until stabilization of vision is recommended
- Progression of anatomic changes does not necessarily correlate with functional loss

TAMOXIFEN TOXICITY

1. Indications for Tamoxifen Use

- Anti-estrogen used in
  - o Breast carcinoma
  - o Hepatocellular carcinoma

2. Risk Factors for Toxicity

- Toxic dose: >180 mg/day
- Cumulative dose: >10 g
- Toxicity is typically not seen within the first 2 years of drug therapy at recommended dose
- *Note*: concurrent AMD not an absolute contraindication

3. Signs and Symptoms of Toxic Maculopathy from Tamoxifen

- Symptoms: blurry vision, acquired dyschromatopsia
- Signs
  - o White-to-yellow perimacular refractile bodies
  - o An acute form manifesting as venous thromboembolic signs has also been described
  - o Patients may also present with normal appearing fundus and unexplained vision loss or no symptoms

- ▪ Characteristic SD-OCT abnormality is diagnostic — see below.

- o Other associated findings: cystoid macular edema (CME), Posterior sub capsular cataract

4. Major Differential Diagnosis for Toxic Crystalline Retinopathy

- Nitrofurantoin
- Canthaxanthine
- Methoxyflurane
- Talc

5. Diagnostic Tests

- Fluorescein angiography

  - o May be needed rule out other etiologies
  - o Associated CME may be angiographic or non-angiographic

- SD-OCT can be used for screening or diagnosis

  - o Characteristic microcystic changes within the central macula with focal patches of photoreceptor disruption and abnormality may be seen without any associated fundus or fluorescein abnormalities (Figure 2)
  - o CME may be present

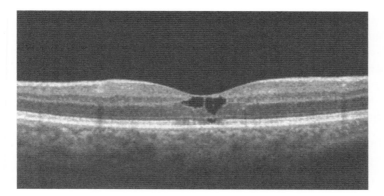

Figure 2. Spectral-domain OCT imaging of the macula of an asymptomatic patient on tamoxifen therapy for four years for breast cancer showing early signs of toxicity. This patient had normal appearing fundus and fluorescein angiography.

6. Management

- Discussion with oncologist the option of stopping the drug
- Anti-vascular endothelial growth factor therapy or intra vitreal steroid can be tried to treat any associated CME

7. Follow-up and Prognosis

- Normal fundus and OCT

  o Baseline examination followed by fundus exam and OCT every 2 years

- Resulting structural and functional photoreceptor abnormality may be irreversible

References

1. Olsen NJ, Schleich MA, Karp DR. Multifaceted effects of hydroxychloroquine in human disease. *Semin Arthritis Rheum* 2013;43(2):264–272.
2. Melles RB, Marmor MF. The risk of toxic retinopathy in patients on long-term hydroxychloroquine therapy. *JAMA Ophthalmol* 2014;3459.
3. Tehrani R, Ostrowski RA, Hariman R, *et al.* Ocular toxicity of hydroxychloroquine. *Semin Ophthalmol* 2008;23(3):201–209.
4. Mittra RA, Mieler WF. Drug toxicity of the posterior segment. In Retina textbook, SJ Ryan, 5th edn., Mosby (Maryland, US) 2013;89:1532–1547.
5. Retrieved from http://www.aao.org/publications/eyenet/201106/pearls.cfm?Render ForPrint=1&, (Last accessed on May 18, 2014).
6. Chen E, Brown DM, Benz MS, *et al.* Spectral domain optical coherence tomography as an effective screening test for hydroxychlororquine retinopathy. *Clin Ophthalmol* 2010;21(4):1151–1158.
7. Marmor MF, Carr RE, Easterbrook M, *et al.* American Academy of Ophthalmology. Recommendations on screening for chloroquine and hydroxychloroquine retinopathy: A report by the American academy of ophthalmology. *Ophthalmol* 2002;109(7): 1377–1382.
8. Marmor MF, Kellner U, Lai TY, *et al.* American Academy of Ophthalmology. Revised recommendations on screening for chloroquine and hydroxychloroquine retinopathy. *Ophthalmol* 2011;118(2):415–422.
9. Marmor MF. Is thioridazine retinopathy progressive? Relationship of pigmentary changes to visual function. *Br J Ophthalmol* 1990;74(12):739–742.
10. Gorin MB, Day R, Costantino JP, *et al.* Long-term tamoxifen citrate use and potential ocular toxicity. *Am J Ophthalmol* 1998;125(4):493–501.
11. Park SS, Zawadzki RJ, Truong SN, *et al.* Microcystoid maculopathy associated with tamoxifen diagnosed by Fourier-domain high resolution optical coherence tomography. *Retinal Cases & Brief Reports* 2009;3(1):33–35.

SECTION 3:
RETINAL VASCULAR
DISORDER

Chapter 9: Proliferative Diabetic Retinopathy

Sumeer Thinda and Susanna S. Park

1. Incidence of Proliferative Diabetic Retinopathy (PDR)

a. There is 6.96% incidence of PDR among those with Diabetes Mellitus (DM)
b. Incidence strongly correlated with duration and type of DM

  i. Type 1 DM: 25% with PDR after 15 years of DM
  56% with PDR after >20 years of DM
  ii. Type 2 DM: 20% with PDR for DM >15 years if taking insulin
  4% with PDR for DM >15 years if not taking insulin

2. Clinical Features

a. Bilateral usually: If asymmetric, consider concurrent ocular ischemic syndrome or retinal vein occlusion in more severe eye or loss of vision from macular scar or optic neuropathy in less severe eye
b. Retinal neovascularization of the disc or elsewhere with retinal dot-blot hemorrhages and microaneurysms: look for high risk features since Diabetic Retinopathy Study (DRS) showed >50% reduction in severe vision loss with Pan Retinal Laser (PRP) over 5 years for eyes with high risk characteristics:

  - Neovascularization of the Disc (NVD) >1/4 disc area
  - Any size NVD with Vitreous Hemorrhage (VH)
  - Neovascularization elsewhere (NVE) > ½ disc area with VH

73

c. Tractional Retinal Detachment (TRD): (Figure 1)

   i. May not be symptomatic till macula becomes involved

   ii. Macular striae may suggest early macular traction

d. Neovascularization of the iris or angle leading to glaucoma.

e. Pregnancy can be associated with worsening of retinopathy, but for some, regression of retinopathy occurs after delivery

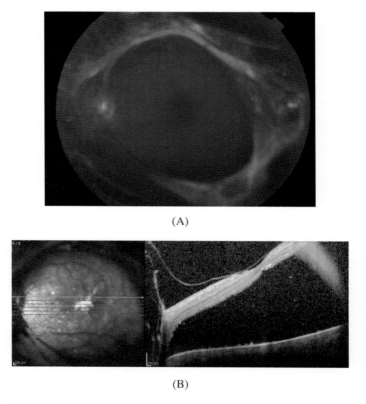

(A)

(B)

Figure 1. Tractional retinal detachment in a table-top configuration. (A) Fundus photograph showing fibrovascular tissue along the superior and inferior arcades with a macula involving TRD with associated macular striae. (B) Macular OCT images demonstrate the table-top configuration and macula-involvement of the TRD (Courtesy of Ala Moshiri, University of California Davis Eye Center).

3. Diagnostic Testing

a. Usually not necessary since diagnosis can be made on clinical examination
b. Fluorescein angiogram indications:

    i. Confirm diagnosis of diabetic retinopathy in atypical cases
    ii. Confirm presence of retinal neovascularization or ischemia if neovascularization is not seen on examination

c. OCT of macula

    i. To screen for possible associated diabetic macular edema before PRP
    ii. To evaluate for macula involvement of TRD (Figure 1)

d. B-scan ultrasonography:

    i. To evaluate for retinal detachment through media opacity
    ii. To evaluate for tractional retinal elevation (Figure 2)

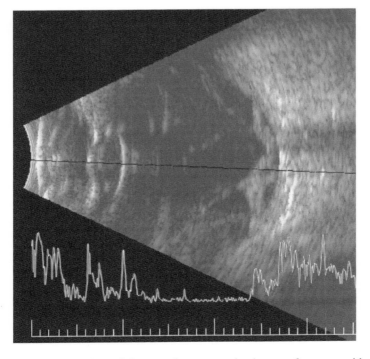

Figure 2. Macular horizontal B-scan ultrasonography image of an eye with severe proliferative diabetic retinopathy and vitreous hemorrhage showing multiple dense tractional epiretinal membranes with associated with TRD involving the macula.

4. Differential Diagnosis

Radiation retinopathy
Retinal vein occlusion
Ocular ischemic syndrome
Eales' disease

5. Management

a. Control modifiable risk factors: hyperglycemia, hypertension, hyperlipidemia, obesity
b. Scatter PRP for high-risk PDR or NVI/NVA (Table 1)

  i. Types of delivery

    1. Slit lamp biomicroscopy: Better focus and control
    2. Pattern laser: Faster and improved patients comfort but not all laser spots might have equal uptake
    3. Indirect laser: Ideal for supplemental laser or laser through media opacity, since more peripheral retina can be treated

  ii. Laser wavelength

    1. **Argon:** Green, 532 nm

      a. Most commonly used
      b. Absorbed by melanin and hemoglobin

    2. **Yellow:** 561 nm

      a. Peak hemoglobin absorption but minimal xanthophyll absorption
      b. Less scatter, better comfort
      c. Good penetration through cataract and old VH

Table 1. Pan retinal laser photocoagulation settings.

Spot size (μm)	200–500
Duration (sec)	0.02–0.20
Burn separation	½–1 burn width apart
Visible endpoint	Gray-white burn
Location	Start with inferior periphery, then treat superiorly
	Avoid long posterior ciliary nerves
	Treat all areas of known non perfusion based on FA
Wavelength	Green, Red, Yellow, Diode

3. **Red:** 670 nm

    a. Less hemoglobin absorption and scatter

    b. Good penetration through fresh VH

iii. Extent of PRP

1. DRS protocol is to treat all peripheral retina outside the temporal arcade
2. Modified protocol: To treat only peripheral ischemic retina as visualized by fluorescein angiography

    a. May minimize complications associated with PRP

    b. Relative efficacy of this modified protocol compared to the DRS protocol for PRP is yet to be determined

iv. Complications of PRP

1. Decreased night vision
2. Constriction of peripheral visual field
3. Temporary loss of accommodation
4. Worsening of macular edema
5. Choroidal effusion

c. Intravitreal Anti-Vascular endothelial growth factor (VEGF) Therapy

i. Bevacizumab (Avastin) Indications:

1. Iris Neovascularization (NVI) and/or Neovascular Glaucoma (NVG)

    a. Rapid regression of NVI within a few days may be noted

i. Rapid regression of NVI may help control Intra Ocular Pressure (IOP) associated with early NVG where the angle is still open

ii. Not effective in controlling IOP in patients with advanced NVG and closed angle

    b. Used in acute management until PRP is administered.

    c. Contralateral eye response has been reported

2. Pretreatment prior to vitrectomy to decrease intraoperative or postoperative vitreous hemorrhage

    a. Applied within 5–7 days of vitrectomy

    b. May worsen tractional retinal detachment which typically occurs 3–31 days after bevacizumab injection, mean 13 days

ii. May be used to treat associated diabetic macular edema before PRP

    iii. Not indicated for management of PDR or associated vitreous hemorrhage.

        1. No long-term visual benefit although vitreous hemorrhage may clear faster

d. Pars plana vitrectomy

  1. Indications

    a. Non clearing vitreous hemorrhage

    b. Macula involving or threatening tractional retinal detachment

  2. Advantages of vitrectomy

    a. Improved control of PDR

        i. Intraoperative PRP administered after removal of associated vitreous hemorrhage allows a more complete PRP to be administered

        ii. PRP can be administered to the ischemic and detached peripheral retina in cases of tractional retinal detachment

        iii. Posterior hyaloid face removal may eliminate scaffold for recurrent retinal NV growth

        iv. Improved intravitreal oxygen level may be beneficial for the ischemic retina

    b. Visual benefit

        i. Faster visual improvement possible from removal of associated vitreous hemorrhage

        ii. Repair of tractional retinal detachment may improve vision and/or minimize risk of further vision loss from increasing macular involvement of traction retinal detachment

    c. Limitations

        i. Risks inherent to vitrectomy

            1. Cataract progression in phakic eyes

            2. Recurrent vitreous hemorrhage

            3. Rhegmatogenous retinal detachment

            4. Endophthalmitis

        ii. Risk of anesthesia since these patients have concurrent cardiovascular risk factors

6. Follow-up Recommendations

a. Active PDR with NVI

   i. 1–4 weeks to check IOP and evaluate response to treatment

b. Active PDR without NVI or vitreous hemorrhage

   i. 1–3 months to evaluate response to treatment

c. PDR with new vitreous hemorrhage

   i. 2–4 weeks to rule out retinal tear or detachment and administer PRP once vitreous hemorrhage clears

d. Inactive PDR

   i. 3–6 months

e. Pregnancy

   i. Initial examination in the 1st trimester, then every 1–3 months

References

1. Yau JW, Rogers SL, Kawasaki R, *et al*. Global prevalence and major risk factors of diabetic retinopathy. *Diabetes Care* 2012;35(3):556–564.
2. Ding J, Wong TY. Current epidemiology of diabetic retinopathy and diabetic macular edema. *Curr Diab Rep* 2012;12(4):346–354.
3. Cheung N, Wong TY. Diabetic retinopathy and systemic vascular complications. *Prog Retin Eye Res* 2008;27(2):161–176.
4. Davis MD, Fisher MR, Gangnon RE, *et al*. Risk factors for high-risk proliferative diabetic retinopathy and severe visual loss: Early Treatment Diabetic Retinopathy Study Report #18. *Invest Ophthalmol Vis Sci* 1998;39(2):233–252.
5. Early photocoagulation for diabetic retinopathy. ETDRS report number 9. Early Treatment Diabetic Retinopathy Study Research Group. *Ophthalmol* 1991;98 (5 Suppl):766–785.
6. Photocoagulation treatment of proliferative diabetic retinopathy. Clinical application of Diabetic Retinopathy Study (DRS) findings, DRS Report Number 8. The Diabetic Retinopathy Study Research Group. *Ophthalmol* 1981;88(7):583–600.
7. Bhatnagar A, Ghauri AJ, Hope-Ross M, *et al*. Diabetic retinopathy in pregnancy. *Curr Diabetes Rev* 2009;5(3):151–156.
8. Mainster MA. Wavelength selection in macular photocoagulation. Tissue optics, thermal effects, and laser systems. *Ophthalmol* 1986;93(7):952–958.
9. Muqit MM, Marcellino GR, Henson DB, *et al*. Optos-guided pattern scan laser (Pascal)-targeted retinal photocoagulation in proliferative diabetic retinopathy. *Acta Ophthalmol* 2013;91(3):251–258.
10. Wakabayashi T, Oshima Y, Sakaguchi H, *et al*. Intravitreal bevacizumab to treat iris neovascularization and neovascular glaucoma secondary to ischemic retinal diseases in 41 consecutive cases. *Ophthalmol* 2008;115(9):1571–1580, 1580 e1571–1573.
11. Ababneh OH, Yousef YA, Gharaibeh AM, *et al*. Intravitreal bevacizumab in the treatment of diabetic ocular neovascularization. *Retina* 2013;33(4):748–755.
12. Zhao LQ, Zhu H, Zhao PQ, *et al*. A systematic review and meta-analysis of clinical outcomes of vitrectomy with or without intravitreal bevacizumab pretreatment for severe diabetic retinopathy. *Br J Ophthalmol* 2011;95(9):1216–1222.
13. Torres-Soriano ME, Reyna-Castelan E, Hernandez-Rojas M, *et al*. Tractional retinal detachment after intravitreal injection of bevacizumab in proliferative diabetic retinopathy. *Retinal cases & brief reports* 2009;3(1):70–73.
14. Cho WB, Oh SB, Moon JW, *et al*. Panretinal photocoagulation combined with intravitreal bevacizumab in high-risk proliferative diabetic retinopathy. *Retina* 2009; 29(4):516–522.
15. Diabetic Retinopathy Clinical Research N. Randomized clinical trial evaluating intravitreal ranibizumab or saline for vitreous hemorrhage from proliferative diabetic retinopathy. *JAMA ophthalmol* 2013;131(3):283–293.

16. Bressler SB, Qin H, Melia M, *et al.* Exploratory analysis of the effect of intravitreal ranibizumab or triamcinolone on worsening of diabetic retinopathy in a randomized clinical trial. *JAMA ophthalmol* 2013;131(8):1033–1040.

17. Avery RL, Pearlman J, Pieramici DJ, *et al.* Intravitreal bevacizumab (Avastin) in the treatment of proliferative diabetic retinopathy. *Ophthalmol* 2006;113:1695–1705.

18. Smiddy WE, Flynn HW, Jr. Vitrectomy in the management of diabetic retinopathy. *Survey of ophthalmology* 1999;43(6):491–507.

19. Arevalo JF, Maia M, Flynn Jr. HW, *et al.* Tractional retinal detachment following intravitreal bevacizumab (Avastin) in patients with severe proliferative diabetic retinopathy. *Br J Ophthalmol* 2008;92(2):213–216.

Chapter 10: Diabetic Macular Edema

Sumeer Thinda, Lawrence S. Morse and Susanna S. Park

1. Incidence of Diabetic Macular Edema (DME)

a. 6 to 13% overall among all with diabetes mellitus (DM)
b. 20 to 30% prevalence among those with DM for more than 20 years

    i. Strongly correlated with duration of DM

2. Factors Associated with Severity of DME

a. Duration of DM
b. Hemoglobin A1c
c. Severity of diabetic retinopathy
d. Type of DM
e. Concurrent hypertension
f. Hyperlipidemia
g. Fluid retention
h. Hypoalbuminemia

3. Clinical Features of DME

a. Usually bilateral but can be asymmetric
b. Defined as edema within 2 disc diameter from fovea associated with retinal microvascular abnormalities (exudates, microaneurysms)
c. May be diffuse or focal

d. Visual acuity decreased as edema involves the fovea or macular ischemia occurs.
e. Clinically significant macular edema (CSME) is criteria for macular laser (Early Treatment of Diabetic Retinopathy Study (ETDRS))

    i. Diagnosed based on biomicroscopy findings, not on ancillary imaging
    ii. Definition based on ETDRS

        1. Thickening of the retina at or within 500 μm of the center of the macula
        2. Hard exudates at or within 500 μm of the center of the macula with adjacent thickening of the retina
        3. Retinal thickening 1 disc area or larger located within 1 disc diameter of the center of the macula

4. Diagnostic Testing

a. Optical Coherence Tomography (OCT)

    i. Good screening tool for DME
    ii. May be more sensitive than biomicroscopy in detecting edema
    iii. Associated subretinal fluid may be visualized in severe cases (15%)
    iv. Associated intraretinal exudates are seen as hyper-reflective intraretinal deposits
    v. Macular thickness map allow quantitation of macular edema
    vi. Allow visualization of vitreomacular traction or epiretinal membrane that may contribute to macular edema

b. Fluorescein angiogram

    i. Important for determining the etiology of macular edema if diagnosis of DME cannot be made on clinical examination
    ii. Microvascular abnormalities (usually microaneurysms) are seen causing late macular leakage

        1. Leakage may be focal or diffuse
        2. Leaking microaneurysms may be better visualized for focal macular laser treatment

    iii. Macular perfusion can be evaluated by visualizing the foveal avascular zone (FAZ)

        1. Best visualized during A/V transit phase of angiography
        2. Enlargement or irregularity of FAZ would suggest macular ischemia

5. Differential Diagnosis of DME

a. Macular edema associated with other retinal vascular abnormality

    i. Retinal vein occlusion, radiation retinopathy, Coat's disease, macroaneurysm

b. Pseudophakic cystoid macular edema
c. Non leaking cystoid macular edema

    i. Niacin, retinitis pigmentosa, Goldmann–Favre syndrome, paclitaxel

d. Macular telangiectasia
e. Macular schisis
f. Macular pucker and associated macular edema or schisis
g. Vitreo-macular traction

6. Management of DME

a. Modify associated risk factors

    i. Hyperglycemia, hypertension, hyperlipidemia, obesity, fluid retention, medications

b. Macula Laser Photocoagulation

    i. Indications: update of ETDRS indications in anti-vascular endothelial growth factor (VEGF) era

        1. CSME not involving fovea without macular ischemia
        2. CSME with foveal involvement when other therapies are not options (e.g. pregnancy)
        3. CSME with foveal involvement when combined with intravitreal anti-VEGF or corticosteroid therapy

    ii. Advantages

        1. Longer duration of action than intravitreal drug therapy
        2. No systemic risk
        3. No risk of intraocular bleeding or infection

    iii. Disadvantages

        1. Macular scar which may leading to scotoma or choroidal neovascularization or scar enlarge on follow-up
        2. Submacular fibrosis which may limit vision
        3. Potential to worsen macular ischemia and vision

4. Delay in macular edema resolution compared to intravitreal drug therapy may lead to less optimum visual outcome

iv. Types of Laser Application Methods (Table 1)

Table 1. Types of macular laser application for DME.

	ETDRS*	mETDRS**	SDM#
Focal Treatment			
Spot size (μm)	50–100	50	N/A
Duration (sec)	≤ 0.10	0.05–0.10	
Visible Endpoint	Definite whitening or darkening of MA	Change in MA color not required, should have at least mild gray burn underneath all MA	
Location	Treat all leaking MA 500–3000 μm from center of macula (but not within 500 μm of disc)	Treat all leaking MA 500–3000 μm from center of macula (but not within 500 μm of disc)	
Grid Treatment			
Spot size (μm)	50–200	50	200
Duration (sec)	≤ 0.10	0.05–0.10	0.20
Burn separation	1 burn width apart	2 burn widths apart	Confluent
Visible Endpoint	Light to moderate intensity	Barely visible	Invisible
Location	Treat all areas of diffuse leakage or non-perfusion within 500–3000 μm from center of macula (but not within 500 μm of disc)	Treat all areas of diffuse leakage or non-perfusion within 500–3000 μm from center of macula except temporally where 500–3500 μm is treated (but not within 500 μm of disc)	Treat entire region (including unthickened retina) within 500–3000 μm from center of macula except temporally where 500–3500 μm is treated (but not within 500 μm of disc)
Wavelength	Green to yellow	Green to yellow	Green to yellow

*ETDRS: conventional laser application method as outlined by ETDRS (Early Treatment of Diabetic Retinopathy Study).
** mETDRS: modification to the laser application outlined in ETDRS commonly applied.
#SDM: subthreshold diode micropulse laser.
MA: microaneurysm.

     1. EDTRS laser method: conventional
     2. mETDRS laser: modified laser application
     3. Subthreshold diode micropulse (SDM) laser

c. Intravitreal Anti-VEGF therapy

  i. Indications

     1. DME with central involvement with visual acuity 20/30 or worse

  ii. Advantages

     1. Lower risk of cataract or glaucoma compared to intravitreal corticosteroids
     2. No permanent laser-induced macular scar
     3. Possible improvement in severity of retinopathy
     4. Better visual outcome than macular laser alone for center involving DME
     5. Potential effect on contralateral eye

  iii. Disadvantages

     1. Shorter duration of action than intravitreal corticosteroid or macular laser
     2. Risk of worsening traction retinal detachment
     3. Contraindicated in pregnant females
     4. Potential systemic risk

  iv. Anti-VEGF agents available (Table 2)

     1. Ranibizumab (Lucentis) 0.3 mg/0.5 cc: FDA approved
     2. Aflibercept (Eylea) 2 mg/0.5 cc: FDA
     3. Bevacizumab (Avastin) 1.25 mg/0.5 cc: off-label use since 2005

d. Intravitreal Corticosteroid Therapy

  i. Indication

     1. DME with central involvement in pseudophakic eyes without glaucoma
     2. DME with central involvement refractory to other therapies
     3. Can be used combined with macular laser

  ii. Advantages

     1. Longer duration of action than anti-VEGF therapy
     2. Less risk of progression of tractional retinal detachment than anti-VEGF therapy

Table 2. Anti-VEGF agents for DME.

Anti-VEGF Agent	Clinical Study	Clinical Study Summary
Ranibizumab (Lucentis)	RESOLVE	Ranibizumab was superior to sham injections (with rescue conventional laser) at 1 year.
	READ-2	Combination therapy with ranibizumab and conventional laser required less ranibizumab injections and resulted in more resolution of macular edema compared to ranibizumab monotherapy at 2 years.
	RESTORE	Ranibizumab monotherapy and combination therapy with conventional laser were both superior to only conventional laser at 1 year.
	DRCR.net Protocol I	Ranibizumab may be more effective than triamcinolone acetonide with fewer side effects. Ranibizumab with deferred conventional laser was superior to ranibizumab with prompt conventional laser at 3 years.
	RISE/RIDE	Ranibizumab 0.3 mg and 0.5 mg were both superior to sham injections (with rescue conventional laser) at 3 years. Delay in treatment may result in poorer visual outcomes.
Bevacizumab (Avastin)	BOLT	Bevacizumab was superior to conventional laser at 2 years.
Aflibercept (Eylea)	DA VINCI	Aflibercept 2 mg q4 weeks was most effective (compared to 0.5 mg q4 weeks, 3 initial monthly doses of 2 mg followed by every 8 weeks, and 3 initial monthly doses of 2 mg followed by PRN) at 1 year.
	VISTA/VIVID	Aflibercept 2 mg q4 weeks was similar to 5 initial monthly doses of 2 mg followed by every 8 weeks at 1 year. Both groups were superior to conventional laser.

    3. Can be used in pregnant females

    4. May be treatment of choice when concurrent inflammatory CME is present

  iii. Disadvantages

    1. Risk of cataract and glaucoma

  iv. Intravitreal corticosteroid agents available for DME (Table 3)

    1. Triamcinolone acetonide (1mg most often used dose)

      a. Triesence (FDA approved); Kenalog (off-label)

      b. Duration of action: average 3 months

Table 3.   Corticosteroids for DME.

Corticosteroid	Clinical Study	Clinical Study Summary
Triamcinolone acetonide (Triesence)	DRCR.net Protocol B	Conventional laser alone was superior with fewer side effects than with either 1mg or 4mg triamcinolone acetonide alone at 2 years. Of note, patients were evaluated every 4 months and potentially undertreated with triamincolone.
	DRCR.net Protocol I	Combination therapy with triamcinolone acetonide and prompt conventional laser was similar to intravitreal ranibizumab in pseudophakic eyes at 2 years although it was associated with higher incidence of adverse effects (cataracts and elevated IOP).
Dexamethasone implant (Ozurdex)	MEAD	Dexamethasone 0.7 mg and 0.35 mg were both superior to sham injections and laser at 3 years but were associated with increased incidence of cataracts and elevated IOP.
Fluocinolone acetonide implant (Iluvien)	FAME	Fluocinolone acetonide (releasing 0.2 μg/day or 0.5 μg/day) were superior to sham injection at 3 years. Greatest benefit was seen in patients with chronic DME (defined as DME for more than 3 years) although there was a high incidence of cataracts and elevated IOP.

2. Dexamethasone implant (Ozurdex)

   a. FDA approved for DME
   b. Duration of action: 4 to 6 months
   c. Contraindicated in aphakic eyes or pseudophakic eyes without an intact lens capsule

3. Fluocinolone acetonide implant (Iluvien 190 μg intravitreal)

   a. FDA approved for DME
   b. Duration of action: up to 3 years

v. Pars planar vitrectomy

   1. Indication: DME refractory all other therapy with associated vitreo-macular traction or epiretinal membrane
   2. DRCR (Diabetic Retinopathy Clinic Research) Network Study of pars plana vitrectomy (PPV) for DME

      a. 43% had improved DME after PPV
      b. 38% had improved visual acuity after PPV
      c. 22% had worsened visual acuity after PPV

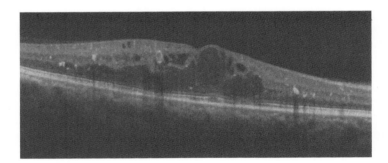

Figure 1. DME. OCT showing hyperreflective exudates and cystoid macular edema involving the foveal center.

References

1. Yau JW, Rogers SL, Kawasaki R, *et al*. Global prevalence and major risk factors of diabetic retinopathy. *Diabetes Care* 2012;35(3):556–564.
2. Ding J, Wong TY. Current epidemiology of diabetic retinopathy and diabetic macular edema. *Curr Diab Rep* 2012;12(4):346–354.
3. Cheung N, Wong TY. Diabetic retinopathy and systemic vascular complications. *Prog Retin Eye Res* 2008;27(2):161–176.
4. Photocoagulation for diabetic macular edema. Early Treatment Diabetic Retinopathy Study Report Number 1. Early Treatment Diabetic Retinopathy Study Research Group. *Arch Ophthalmol* 1985;103(12):1796–1806.
5. Bressler NM, Miller KM, Beck RW, *et al*. Observational study of subclinical diabetic macular edema. *Eye* 2012;26(6):833–840.
6. Kylstra JA, Brown JC, Jaffe GJ, *et al*. The importance of fluorescein angiography in planning laser treatment of diabetic macular edema. *Ophthalmol* 1999;106(11):2068–2073.
7. Dmuchowska DA, Krasnicki P, Mariak Z. Can optical coherence tomography replace fluorescein angiography in detection of ischemic diabetic maculopathy? *Graefes Arch Clin Exp Ophthalmol* 2014;252(5):731–738.
8. Fong DS, Strauber SF, Aiello LP, *et al*. Comparison of the modified early treatment diabetic retinopathy study and mild macular grid laser photocoagulation strategies for diabetic macular edema. *Arch Ophthalmol* 2007;125(4):469–480.
9. Schatz H, Madeira D, McDonald HR, *et al*. Progressive enlargement of laser scars following grid laser photocoagulation for diffuse diabetic macular edema. *Arch Ophthalmol* 1991;109(11):1549–1551.
10. Fong DS, Segal PP, Myers F, *et al*. Subretinal fibrosis in diabetic macular edema. ETDRS report 23. Early Treatment Diabetic Retinopathy Study Research Group. *Arch Ophthalmol* 1997;115(7):873–877.
11. Lavinsky D, Cardillo JA, Melo LA, Jr., *et al*. Randomized clinical trial evaluating mETDRS versus normal or high-density micropulse photocoagulation for diabetic macular edema. *Invest Ophthalmol Vis Sci* 2011;52(7):4314–4323.
12. Massin P, Bandello F, Garweg JG, *et al*. Safety and efficacy of ranibizumab in diabetic macular edema (RESOLVE Study): A 12-month, randomized, controlled, double-masked, multicenter phase II study. *Diabetes Care* 2010;33(11):2399–2405.
13. Nguyen QD, Shah SM, Khwaja AA, *et al*. Two-year outcomes of the ranibizumab for edema of the macula in diabetes (READ-2) study. *Ophthalmol* 2010;117(11):2146–2151.
14. Mitchell P, Bandello F, Schmidt-Erfurth U, *et al*. The RESTORE study: Ranibizumab monotherapy or combined with laser versus laser monotherapy for diabetic macular edema. *Ophthalmol* 2011;118(4):615–625.

15. Elman MJ, Bressler NM, Qin H, *et al*. Expanded 2-year follow-up of ranibizumab plus prompt or deferred laser or triamcinolone plus prompt laser for diabetic macular edema. *Ophthalmol* 2011;118(4):609–614.

16. Elman MJ, Qin H, Aiello LP, *et al*. Intravitreal ranibizumab for diabetic macular edema with prompt versus deferred laser treatment: Three-year randomized trial results. *Ophthalmol* 2012;119(11):2312–2318.

17. Brown DM, Nguyen QD, Marcus DM, *et al*. Long-term outcomes of ranibizumab therapy for diabetic macular edema: the 36-month results from two phase III trials: RISE and RIDE. *Ophthalmol* 2013;120(10):2013–2022.

18. Rajendram R, Fraser-Bell S, Kaines A, *et al*. A 2-year prospective randomized controlled trial of intravitreal bevacizumab or laser therapy (BOLT) in the management of diabetic macular edema: 24-month data: report 3. *Arch Ophthalmol* 2012;130(8):972–979.

19. Do DV, Nguyen QD, Boyer D, *et al*. One-year outcomes of the da Vinci Study of VEGF Trap-Eye in eyes with diabetic macular edema. *Ophthalmol* 2012;119(8): 1658–1665.

20. Korobelnik JF, Do DV, Schmidt-Erfurth U, *et al*. Intravitreal aflibercept for diabetic macular edema. *Ophthalmol* 2014.

21. Ip MS, Bressler SB, Antoszyk AN, *et al*. A randomized trial comparing intravitreal triamcinolone and focal/grid photocoagulation for diabetic macular edema: Baseline features. *Retina* 2008;28(7):919–930.

22. Campochiaro PA, Brown DM, Pearson A, *et al*. Sustained delivery fluocinolone acetonide vitreous inserts provide benefit for at least 3 years in patients with diabetic macular edema. *Ophthalmol* 2012;119(10):2125–2132.

23. Boyer DS, Yoon YH, Belfort R, Jr., *et al*. Three-year, randomized, sham-controlled trial of dexamethasone intravitreal implant in patients with diabetic macular edema. *Ophthalmol* 2014;121(10):1904–1914.

24. Diabetic Retinopathy Clinical Research Network Writing Committee on behalf of the DRCR.net. Visual outcome in eyes with diabetic macular edema and vitreomacular traction. *Ophthlamol* 2010;117:1087–1093.

Chapter 11: Retinal Vein Occlusion

Susanna S. Park

1. Incidence

180,000 eyes/year in USA

- 2nd most common retinal vascular cause of vision loss
- 5th most common cause of unilateral vision loss in the elderly

2. Types

- Central Retinal Vein Occlusion (CRVO)
- Branch Retinal Vein Occlusion (BRVO)

  o Supratemporal (60%); Infratemporal (40%)

- Hemiretinal Vein Occlusion (HemiRVO)

  o Considered subclass of CRVO or BRVO

3. Risk Factors

- Common: age (>55 years, mean 65 years), hypertension (50–70%), cardiovascular disease, diabetes mellitus, increased body mass index
- Rare associations

  o Hypercoagulable or hyperviscosity states
  o Vasculitis: syphilis, sarcoidosis, collagen vascular disease, etc.
  o Optic nerve drusen
  o External compression: increased intraorbital pressure

4. Clinical Presentation

- Acute painless unilateral loss of vision or visual field defect

  o 5% bilateral but not simultaneous
  o Occasional history of transient visual blurring
  o Presenting visual acuity: 20/20 to Hand Motions
  o Possible afferent pupillary defect in severe cases

- Fundus Findings

  o Acute findings

    ▪ Retinal Hemorrhages, dilated tortuous veins, cotton wool spots, disc edema
    ▪ BRVO: quadrant or wedge-shaped sector involvement radiating from an arteriovenous crossing site
    ▪ CRVO: all four quadrants involved

  o Chronic findings

    ▪ Macular edema (50%)
    ▪ Collaterals vessels (may not correlate with visual outcome)
    ▪ Neovascularization (Disc, Retina, Iris) with vitreous hemorrhage or neovascular glaucoma

      □ Risk for ischemic CRVO; rare with BRVO

5. Differential Diagnosis

- Diabetic retinopathy: characteristic microaneurysms with dot-blot hemorrhages, usually bilateral without history of acute vision loss unless vitreous hemorrhage
- Venous stasis retinopathy: mid-peripheral blot hemorrhages without history of acute vision loss; may develop iris neovascularization
- Hypertensive retinopathy: flame-shaped hemorrhages with minimal venous congestion; disc edema if severe; often bilateral
- Leukemia: hemorrhages and cotton wool spots with minimal venous congestion
- Anemia: hemorrhages and Roth's spots with minimal venous congestion
- Papillophlebitis: benign variant simulating CRVO in a young patient
- Disc edema/Papilledema: can simulate mild CRVO but disc edema is more prominent than retinal hemorrhages

6. Evaluation and Diagnostic Testing

- Complete ophthalmic and medical history

  o History of glaucoma, diabetes mellitus, hypertension, hyperlipidemia, cardiovascular disease

- o History of birth control pill use, sickle cell disease, deep vein thrombosis or malignancy
- o Family history of cerebrovascular accident, deep vein thrombosis or pulmonary embolism

- Complete eye examination: include intraocular pressure, gonioscopy and dilated ophthalmoscopy
- Optical coherence tomography (OCT): to evaluate for macular edema
- Check blood pressure
- Fluorescein angiography: to evaluate for retinal ischemia and confirm diagnosis

- o May be deferred if extensive retinal hemorrhages are present
- o Delay in retinal venous filling may be variable depending on severity
- o Evaluate degree of capillary non-perfusion to determine if ischemic RVO

- ■ Ischemic BRVO: ≥5 disc areas non-perfusion
- ■ Ischemic CRVO: ≥10 disc area non-perfusion

- o Evaluate for early leakage from retinal neovascularization and late leakage from cystoid macular edema (Figure 1)

- Laboratory testing

- o Usually done if patient has no known common risk factors for RVO or presents with bilateral or multiple RVO
- o Fasting blood glucose or hemoglobin A1c; lipid profile
- o Complete blood count, sedimentation rate, anti-nuclear antibody (ANA), rheumatoid factor (RF), angiotensin converting enzyme (ACE), syphilis serologies, HIV
- o For suspected hypercoagulable state: anti-phospholipid antibody, lupus anti-coagulant, anti-cardiolipin antibody, protein C and S, homocysteine level, prothrombin/partial thromboplastin time (PT/PTT), serum electrophoresis

---→

Figure 1. (*Figure on facing page*) Fluorescein angiogram of an eye with acute central retinal vein occlusion. (A) Red-free fundus photography showing dilated tortous retinal veins with scattered retinal hemorrhages. (B) Mid-transit fluorescein angiogram of the periphery showing peripheral non-perfusion and staining of the damaged retinal veins. (C) Late-transit angiogram showing diffuse late petalloid leakage into the macula consistent with cystoid macular edema.

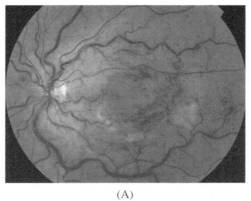

(A)

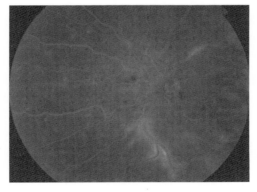

(B)

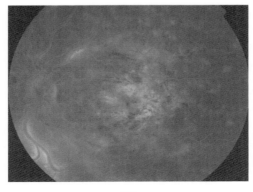

(C)

7. Prognosis

- Causes of vision loss from retinal vein occlusion (RVO)

  o Macular hemorrhage, ischemia and/or edema
  o Late macular fibrosis or pucker (20%)
  o Peripheral retinal ischemia leading to neovascularization and vitreous hemorrhage, tractional retinal detachment and/or neovascular glaucoma

- Ischemic CRVO

  o Typically older patient with poorer presenting vision, afferent pupillary defect and extensive retinal hemorrhages ("blood-and-thunder fundus")
  o Poorer visual prognosis: 90% with visual acuity 20/400 or worse
  o 2/3 risk of neovascular complications at 3 to 5 months after onset

8. Management

- Treat associated medical and/or ophthalmic condition
- Consider aspirin 81 to 325 mg po qd if no medical contraindication
- Followed and treated for macular edema or neovascularization that may be visually significant
- CRVO

  o Evaluate monthly for the first 6 months with gonioscopy and macular OCT, then every 3 to 6 months if stable
  o PRP indications based on the Central Vein Occlusion Study (CVO)

    ▪ Close follow-up and treat for iris neovascularization
    ▪ If poor follow-up expected, consider prophylactic panretinal photocoagulation (PRP) for eyes with capillary non-perfusion >10 disc area since 2/3 are at risk for neovascular complications

  o Macular Edema Treatment for CRVO and HemiRVO

    ▪ Grid macular laser improved edema but not visually beneficial based on CVO Study except for patients <55 years of age
    ▪ Intravitreal Corticosteroid

      □ Triamcinolone: corticosteroid for retinal vein occlusion (SCORE)-CRVO Study (2009)

        — Visual outcome superior to observation

      □ Dexamethasone implant (Ozurdex): GENEVA Study (2009)

        — Visual outcome superior to observation

      □ Risks: cataract and Glaucoma

- Intravitreal anti-vascular endothelial growth factor (VEGF)
  - □ Ranibizumab (Lucentis): FDA approved 2010
    - — Superior to observation: CRUISE Study, 2008
  - □ Aflibercept (Eylea): FDA approved, 2012
    - — Superior to observation: GALILEO and COPERNICUS studies, 2012
  - □ Bevacizumab (Avastin): off-label use since 2005
    - — Level 2 and 3 evidence of superiorly to observation
- o SCORE2 study will compare the relative efficacy of Bevacizumab, Aflibercept and Dexamethasone implant (Ozurdex) for macular edema from CRVO or hemiRVO

- BRVO
  - o Scatter laser indications based on the Branch retinal BVO Study
    - Prophylactic laser not evaluated but not recommended since low risk of visually significant neovascular complications (Iris neovascularization 1%)
    - Observe treat for neovascularization (iris, disc or retina)
    - Vitreous hemorrhage risk decreased from 60 to 30% with scatter laser
  - o Macular edema treatment options
    - Grid laser (BRVO Study, 1984)
      - □ Grid laser treatment superior to observation if foveal avascular zone intact and edema present with VA 20/40 to 20/200 after 3 months
    - Intravitreal corticosteroid
    - Triamcinolone (SCORE: BRVO Study, 2009)
      - □ At 1 and 3 years: grid laser and intravitreal triamcinolone (1 or 4 mg) had equal visual benefit
      - □ 4 mg triamcinolone has higher glaucoma risk
    - Intravitreal Dexamethasone Implant (Ozurdex, FDA approved, 2009)
      - □ Superior visual outcome to Sham injection/grid laser (GENEVA Study)

- o Intravitreal anti-VEGF

  - ▪ Ranibizumab (Lucentis, FDA approved, 2010)

    - □ Superior visual benefit over grid laser (BRVO Study)

  - ▪ Bevacizumab (Avastin, off-label use since 2005)
  - ▪ Used alone or combined with grid laser

- Vitrectomy for RVO

  - o Indications

    - ▪ Non-clearing vitreous hemorrhage
    - ▪ Iris neovascularization with vitreous hemorrhage
    - ▪ Fractional and/or rhegmatogenous retinal detachment
    - ▪ Macular pucker with macular edema resistant to medical therapy

References

1. Brown DM, Campochiora PA, Singh RP, *et al*. Ranibizumab for macular edema following central retinal vein occlusion: Six-month primary end point results of a phase III study. *Ophthalmol* 2010;117:1124–1133.
2. Campochiaro PA, Heier JS, Feiner L, *et al*. Ranibizumab for macular edema following branch retinal vein occlusion: Six-month primary end point results of a phase III study. *Ophthalmol* 2010;117:1102–1112.
3. Hallar JA, Bandello F, Belfort Jr R, *et al*. Ozurdex GENEVA Study Group. Li J. Dexamethasone intravitreal implant in patients with macular edema related to branch or central retinal vein occlusion twelve-month study results. *Ophthalmol* 2011;118: 2453–2460.
4. Ip MS, Scott IU, VanVeldhuisen PC, *et al*. SCORE Study Research Group. A randomized trial comparing the efficacy and safety of intravitreal triamcinolone with observation to treat vision loss associated with macular edema secondary to central retinal vein occlusion: The Standard Care versus. Corticosteroid for Retinal Vein Occlusion (SCORE) Study Report 5. *Arch Ophthalmol* 2009;127:1101–1114.
5. Klein R, Klein BE, Meuer SM. The epidemiology of retinal vein occlusion: the Beaver Dam Eye Study. *Trans Am Ophthalmol Soc* 2000;98:133–141.
6. Scott IU, Ip MS, VanVeldhuisen PC, *et al*. A randomized trial comparing the efficacy and safety of intravitreal triamcinolone with standard care to treat vision loss associated with macular Edema secondary to branch retinal vein occlusion: The Standard Care versus Corticosteroid for Retinal Vein Occlusion (SCORE) Study Report 6. *Arch Ophthalmol* 2009;127:1115–1128.
7. The Branch Vein Occlusion Study Group. Argon laser photocoagulation for macular edema in branch vein occlusion. *Am J Ophthalmol* 1984;98:271–282.
8. The Central Vein Occlusion Study Group. A randomized clinical trial of early panretinal photocoagulation for ischemic central vein occlusion. The Central Vein Occlusion Study Group N report. *Ophthalmology* 1995;102:1434–1444.
9. The Central Vein Occlusion Study Group. Natural history and clinical management of central retinal vein occlusion. *Arch Ophthalmol* 1997;115:486–491.
10. The Eye Disease Case-Control Study Group. Risk factors for central retinal vein occlusion. *Arch Ophthalmol* 1996;114:545–554.

Chapter 12: Retinal Artery Occlusion

Ala Moshiri

Introduction

Retinal artery occlusion usually causes painless permanent vision loss corresponding to the ischemic retina downstream of the occluded vessel. Retinal examination during the acute phases shows slowed blood flow. Sometimes one can see individual red blood cells moving very slowly as a segmented column within the occluded vessel. The affected portion of the retina will appear white due to retinal ganglion cell axonal swelling. In the case of a central retinal artery occlusion (CRAO), the foveal center appears rust–red, a so-called "cherry red spot". This is because there are no ganglion cell axons there to obscure the underlying RPE and choroidal colors. The pallor of the retina lasts 4–6 weeks. The cilioretinal artery (if present) can also become occluded. Isolated cilioretinal artery occlusions usually have a good prognosis. In the case of patients with a cilioretinal artery, central acuity may be spared despite a retinal artery occlusion.

1. Incidence

Estimated at 1 in 100,000

2. Types Based on Location

Branch Retinal Artery Occlusion (BRAO)

— Sectoral vision loss with variable visual acuity

Central Retinal Artery Occlusion (CRAO)

— All four quadrants involved
— Counting Fingers or Hand Motions, unless cilioretinal artery is present

3. Clinical Features

Usually acute painless unilateral vision loss, 1–2% bilateral Associated conditions: ipsilateral carotid artery occlusion, atherosclerosis, cardiac valvular disease, coagulopathies, sickle cell disease, oral contraceptives, homocysteinuria, pregnancy, platelet abnormalities, clotting factor abnormalities, collagen vascular diseases, optic disc drusen, arterial loops, migraine, hypotension, giant cell arteritis

Ethnicity: all
Male > Female
Age of diagnosis: 7th decade of life (patients in their 60's)
Fluorescein or Indocyanine green (ICG) Angiography: delayed arm-to-retinal arterial time
Irreversible retinal cell death occurs within 90 minutes based on animal studies

4. Clinical Findings

a. Anterior Segment Signs

   i. Iris neovascularization (rubeosis iridis)
   ii. Neovascular glaucoma
   iii. Afferent pupillary defect

b. Posterior Segment Signs

   i. Retinal pallor in acute phase leading to "cherry red spot" in CRAO and some BRAO
   ii. Retinal intravascular emboli: variable source

      1. Refractile lesion within the blood vessel (Hollenhorst plaque) is suggestive of carotid disease
      2. A whitish lesion within a section of the blood vessel (platelet fibrin thrombus)
      3. Large calcific plaque is suggestive of cardiac valvular disease

   iii. Narrowed arterioles
   iv. Neovascularization of the disc and elsewhere (up to 20%)
   v. Cilioretinal artery, if present, may allow for improved visual acuity

5. Differential Diagnosis

a. Ophthalmic artery occlusion: no "cherry red spot"
b. Ischemic optic neuropathy

c. Diabetic retinopathy
d. Other retinal vascular disease

6. Diagnostic Testing

a. Baseline imaging

   i. Fundus photography
   ii. Fluorescein angiography: look for delayed retinal vascular filling in acute phase which may normalize during chronic phase
   iii. ICG angiography (look for delayed choroidal filling to distinguish from ophthalmic artery occlusion)
   iv. Optical coherence tomography (OCT) to look for hyperreflective nerve fiber layer during acute phase
   v. Follow-up examination to monitor for neovascularization

      1. May occur within a few weeks of onset of symptoms

b. Electroretinography: both scotopic and photopic recordings will show normal a-wave due to preserved choriodal blood flow, but reduced or absent b-wave due to retinal arterial insufficiency and inner retinal damage (Figure 1)
c. Ophthalmodynamometry: used to estimate the pressure in the ophthalmic artery at the site of origin of the central retinal artery, and is useful to distinguish from ocular ischemic syndrome

7. Management

a. Acute treatment that may be considered

   1. Digital ocular massage
   2. Anterior chamber paracentesis

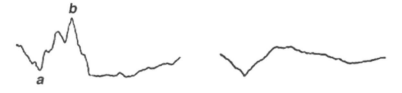

Figure 1.   Electroretinogram (ERG) of a normal eye versus an eye with CRAO. The tracing on the left represents a normal light adapted full-field ERG. The tracing on the right is from an eye that has had a CRAO. The a-wave is normal, but the b-wave is barely above the baseline, and can be absent altogether.

     3.   Glaucoma medications

     4.   Aspirin

     5.   Breathing into a bag to induce vasodilation

b. Chronic treatment is directed toward control of

    i.   Retinal neovascularization via panretinal photocoagulation

    ii. Neovascular glaucoma using a combination of anti-vascular endothelial growth factor (VEGF) therapy, scatter retinal laser, and glaucoma therapy

c. Embolic workup is indicated

    i.   Carotid Doppler Ultrasound

    ii. Echocardiogram

d. Consider Giant Cell Arteritis as cause in elderly

    i.   Order sedimentation rate and C-reactive protein

    ii. Review of systems for associated signs and symptoms:

        1.   Headaches, fever, weight loss, night sweats, jaw claudication, scalp tenderness, proximal muscle weakness

e. Referral to cardiology

f. Lifestyle modifications, cessation of smoking and weight reduction

8. Prognosis

a. In the case of embolic sources, the mortality rate is 56% over 9 years versus an age-matched rate of 27%

References

1. Brown GC, Magargal LE, Shields JA, *et al*. Retinal artery obstruction in children and adults. *Ophthalmol* 1981;88:18–25.
2. Hayreh S, Podhajsky P. Ocular neovascularization with retinal vascular occlusion, II. Occurrence in central and branch retinal artery occlusion. *Arch Ophthalmol* 1982;100:1585–1596.
3. Hayreh SS, Kolder HE, Weingeist TA. Central retinal artery occlusion and retinal tolerance time. *Ophthalmol* 1980;87:75–78.
4. Recchia FM, Brown GC. Systemic disorders associated with retinal vascular occlusion. *Curr Opin Ophthalmol* 2000;11:462–467.
5. Rudkin AK, Lee AW, Chen CS. Ocular neovascularization following central retinal artery occlusion: prevalence and timing of onset. *Eur J Ophthalmol* 2010.
6. Savino PJ, Glaser JS, Cassady J. Retinal stroke: Is the patient at risk? *Arch Ophthalmol* 1977;95:1185–1189.
7. Sharma S, Pater JL, Lam M, *et al*. Can different types of retinal emboli be reliably differentiated from one another? An inter- and intraobserver agreement study. *Can J Ophthalmol* 1998;33:144–148.

Chapter 13: Ocular Ischemic Syndrome

Ala Moshiri

1. Incidence

7.5 cases per million persons per year

2. Clinical Features

Locations: usually unilateral, 22% bilateral
Association: >90% occlusion of ipsilateral carotid artery
Ethnicity: all
Male > Female (2:1)
Age of diagnosis: mean 65 years, rare below age 50
Symptomatic Ocular ischemic syndrome (OIS) in 4% of patients with carotid occlusion

Asymptomatic OIS in 30% of patients with carotid occlusion

— 1.5% of these will become symptomatic per year

Most common symptom is a gradual loss of vision over weeks with or without dull eye ache or headache.

Amaurosis fugax may also occur
Fluorescein or Indocyanine green (ICG) Angiography: delayed arm-to-choroid time

1. Clinical findings

    a. Anterior segment signs

        i. Conjunctival/Episcleral injection

      ii. Corneal edema/hypoesthesia
     iii. Iris atrophy with sluggish pupil
     iv. Iris neovascularization (rubeosis iridis)
      v. Neovascular glaucoma
     vi. Iridocyclitis (cell, flare, keratic precipitates)
    vii. Spontaneous hyphema
   viii. Afferent pupillary defect
     ix. Asymmetric cataract

  b. Posterior segment signs

      i. Narrowed arterioles/Dilated veins
     ii. Retinal hemorrhages (midperipheral retina)
    iii. Microaneurysms
    iv. Telangiectatic vessels
     v. Neovascularization of the disc and elsewhere
    vi. Retinal embolic disease
   vii. Spontaneous pulsations of the central retinal artery
  viii. Anterior ischemic optic neuropathy
    ix. Wedge shaped areas of chorio-retinal atrophy

  c. Orbital signs

      i. Orbital pain is present in 40% of cases

        1. Pain may be ischemic in origin, or due to elevated IOP

     ii. Ophthalmoplegia
    iii. Ptosis

2. Differential diagnosis

  a. Retinal vein occlusion
  b. Retinal artery occlusion
  c. Diabetic retinopathy
  d. Giant cell arteritis
  e. Other retinal vascular disease

3. Management

  a. Baseline imaging

      i. Fundus photography
     ii. Fluorescein angiography (look for delayed retinal vascular filling)

      iii. ICG angiography (look for delayed choroidal filling)

      iv. Consider optical coherence tomography (OCT) to evaluate for retinal thinning and to rule out macular edema associated with simulating conditions

      v. Follow-up examination in few weeks to months depending on severity, associated findings and need for treatment

b. Electroretinography: both scotopic and photopic recordings will show reduced a-wave due to choriodal ischemia, and reduced b-wave due to retinal arterial insufficiency

c. Ophthalmodynamometry: used to estimate the pressure in the ophthalmic artery at the site of origin of the central retinal artery. Measurements are performed by increasing IOP by gradually applying pressure to the globe with a finger on the upper eyelid, while observing the arteries on the optic disc at the slit lamp until they begin to pulsate. The tactile pressure required to produce artery pulsations on the optic disc reflects the ophthalmic artery diastolic pressure, whereas the force required to cause cessation of arterial pulsations reflects the ophthalmic artery systolic pressure

d. Ocular treatment is directed toward control of

      i. Anterior segment inflammation (topical steroids and cycloplegia)

      ii. Retinal ischemia and neovascularization (panretinal photocoagulation)

      iii. Neovascular glaucoma (anti-vascular endothelial growth factor (VEGF) therapy followed by scatter retinal laser and glaucoma therapy)

e. Carotid doppler ultrasound

      i. $\geq 90\%$ stenosis of the ipsilateral carotid arterial system is present in eyes with OIS

f. Carotid angiography

g. Referral to cardiology

      i. The overall mortality rate for patients with OIS is 40% at 5 years with the leading cause of death being cardiovascular disease, usually myocardial infarction, (67%) followed by cerebral infarction. (19%) It is therefore essential that physicians adopt appropriate therapeutic options aiming at primary prevention of myocardial and cerebral infarction, including anti-platelet therapy when indicated

      ii. Carotid endarterectomy, if indicated

      iii. lifestyle modifications, cessation of smoking and weight reduction

References

1. Klijn CJ, Kappelle LJ, van Schooneveld MJ, *et al.* Venous stasis retinopathy in symptomatic carotid artery occlusion: Prevalence, cause, and outcome. *Stroke: A journal of cerebral circulation* 2002;33(3):695–701.
2. Sivalingam A, Brown GC, Magargal LE. The ocular ischemic syndrome. III. Visual prognosis and the effect of treatment. *Int Ophthalmol* 1991;15(1):15–20.
3. Kearns TP, Hollenhorst RW. Venous-stasis retinopathy of occlusive disease of the carotid artery. *Proc staff Meet Mayo Clin* 1963;38:304–312.
4. Mizener JB, Podhajsky P, Hayreh SS. Ocular ischemic syndrome. *Ophthalmol* 1997;104(5):859–864.
5. Sisler HA. A review of ophthalmodynamometry. *Am J Ophthalmol* 1960;50:419–424.

Chapter 14: Retinopathy of Prematurity

Yoshihiro Yonekawa, Benjamin J. Thomas,
Bobeck Modjtahedi, Kimberly A. Drenser, Michael T. Trese
and Antonio Capone Jr.

1. Incidence

1. Cryotherapy for retinopathy of prematurity (CRYO-ROP) (1980s): 66% of screened infants affected by some degree of ROP, and of those, 27% progressed to advanced disease
2. Early treatment for ROP (ETROP) (early 2000s): 68% affected by some degree of ROP, but 37% progressed to advanced disease, owing to more zone 1 disease

2. Who and When to Screen

1. Birth weight (BW) ≤1500 g or gestational age ≤30 weeks
2. Not meeting BW or Gestational age criteria, but unstable course and deemed high-risk by neonatologist
3. First examination: later of either 31 weeks post-menstrual age (PMA) or 4 weeks after delivery. However, we recommend earlier examinations for profoundly premature infants with unstable clinical courses

3. Staging

1. Zones

    1. Zone I: circle centered on optic disc, with radius twice the distance from the disc to the foveal center

    2.   Zone II: anterior edge of zone I to the nasal ora serrate

    3.   Zone III: temporal crescent anterior to zone II

2. Stages (Figures 1–6)

    1.   Immature (termed Stage 0 by some): no demarcation between vascularized and non-vascularized retina

    2.   Stage 1: flat demarcation line

    3.   Stage 2: line is now a ridge with volume

    4.   Stage 3: extraretinal fibrovascular proliferation from the ridge

    5.   Stage 4: retinal detachment (RD) that spares (4A) or involves (4B) the macula

    6.   Stage 5: total RD (open funnel, open-closed, closed-open or closed-closed)

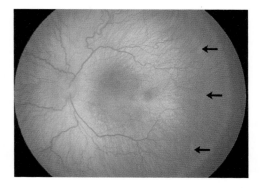

Figure 1. Stage 1 ROP: flat demarcation line between vascular and avascular retina (arrows).

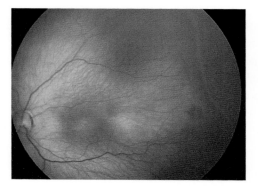

Figure 2. Stage 2 ROP: the demarcation line now is a ridge with volume.

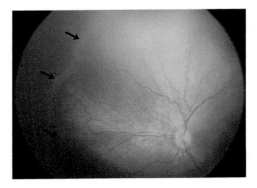

Figure 3. Stage 3 ROP: fibrovascular proliferation from the shunt (arrows).

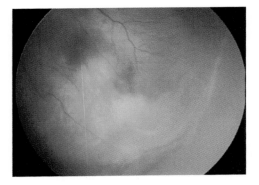

Figure 4. Stage 4A ROP: retinal detachment that does not involve the macula.

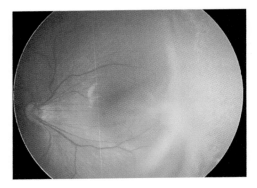

Figure 5. Stage 4B ROP: the detachment involves the macula.

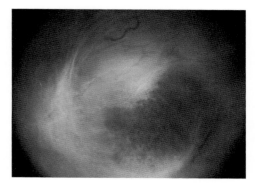

Figure 6. Stage 5 ROP: complete retinal detachment. This patient has an open funnel configuration.

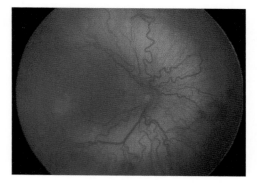

Figure 7. Plus disease: note the vascular dilatation and tortuosity in the posterior pole.

3. Plus Disease (Figure 7)

   1. Plus: vascular dilatation and tortuosity ≥2 quadrants in the posterior pole.
   2. Pre-plus: vascular changes that do not meet criteria for plus

4. Aggressive Posterior ROP (AP-ROP)

   1. Plus disease in zone I or posterior zone II, often with flat neovascularization and rapid progression, which may skip the classic ROP stages? Requires immediate treatment

5. Threshold Disease

    1. 50% risk of progression to RD.

    2. Zone I or II, stage 3 for 5 contiguous or 8 total clock hours, with plus disease.

    3. Was treatment criteria prior to ETROP, but now treatment at Type 1 ROP is the standard of care

6. *Type 1 ROP* (high-risk pre-threshold, >15% RD risk)

    1. Zone I: any stage with plus, or stage 3 without plus

    2. Zone II: stage 2 or 3 with plus

7. *Type 2 ROP* (low-risk pre-threshold, <15% RD risk)

    1. Zone I: stage 1 or 2 without plus

    2. Zone II: stage 3 without plus

4. Follow-up Schedule

1. ≤1 week

    1. Zone I: immature, stage 1 or 2 without plus

    2. Zone II: stage 3 without plus

    3. Any suspicions for AP-ROP

2. 1–2 weeks

    1. Zone I: regressing

    2. Zone II: immature, or stage 2

    3. Evolving telemedicine paradigms employ weekly imaging

3. 2 weeks

    1. Zone II: immature, stage 1, or regressing

4. 2–3 weeks

    1. Zone III: stage 1, 2, or regressing

5. When to conclude screening

    1. Vascularization to zone III and no previous ROP in zone I or II

    2. Full vascularization 360°

    3. PMA 50 weeks with no pre-threshold disease

    4. Regression of ROP with no abnormal tissue that may reactivate

5. Differential Diagnosis

1. Familial exudative vitreoretinopathy
2. Norrie disease
3. Incontinentia pigmenti
4. However, history of prematurity and the clinical appearance supports the diagnosis of ROP in practically all cases

6. Photocoagulation

1. Laser allows control of >90% of Type 1 ROP if performed correctly
2. For Type 2 ROP, wait till progression to Type 1 ROP or threshold disease for laser photocoagulation
3. Laser is superior to cryotherapy in visual outcomes, and causes less myopia
4. Spots should be placed 0.5 to 1 spot-size apart in a near-confluent fashion to the avascular retina from the ridge to the ora, without any skip areas and avoiding ciliary processes and the lens/iris. Red diode laser is recommended. However, potential complications have been reported with both red and green laser use

7. Controversy of Intravitreal Anti-Vascular Endothelial Growth Factor Treatment (VEGF)

1. Laser photocoagulation is the standard of care for ROP treatment
2. We may consider intravitreal bevacizumab if there is poor foveal development and the avascular notch involves the fovea
3. Bevacizumab provides an option to areas without access to laser
4. Early studies indicate that bevacizumab may be effective for zone I disease, but local and systemic complications are not yet known
5. Correct dosing and timing are also unknown
6. If an intravitreal anti-VEGF agent must be used, we recommend using ranibizumab, because it is potentially systemically safer due to shorter half-life and shorter depression of circulating VEGF
7. ROP is the most predictable retinal vascular disease, but bevacizumab alters the biochemistry and follow-up care is undefined due to late reactivation and peripheral vascular abnormalities

8. Surgical Treatment

1. Vitrectomy is the preferred treatment for ROP detachments. Best performed when not vascularly active, to avoid intraoperative hemorrhage. Can laser first to quiet vascular activity

2. Stage 4A: lens-sparing vitrectomy is the treatment of choice, which provides good visual outcomes. Pars plicata incisions are made, and the vitreous is removed to relieve traction. The lens occupies a disproportionately larger volume of the globe and care must be taken to avoid lens-touch
3. Stage 4B: attempts should be made to preserve the lens, but may not be possible if there are membranes on the posterior capsule. Traction is removed by segmenting organized vitreous in the ridge-to-ridge, ridge-to-periphery, ridge-to-lens, and ridge-to-disc vectors. Pre-retinal tissues are firmly attached to the retina and often integrated; it is dangerous to attempt to remove all membranes, because a single iatrogenic break can be the end of the case
4. Stage 5: stage 5 is rare in the U.S. due to widespread knowledge of the CRYO-ROP and ETROP results. Visual prognosis is relatively poor, but intervention can save a child's sight from no light perception to form vision

9. Common Late Sequelae of ROP

1. Myopia
2. Retinal tears and detachments with posterior breaks
3. Strabismus and amblyopia
4. Cataract
5. Closed angle glaucoma
6. Aphakic glaucoma in post-surgical infants requiring lensectomy
7. There are increasing numbers of adult patients with a history of ROP as infants ("adult ROP")

10. Telemedical ROP Screening

1. May improve access to ROP care for the increasing number of premature infants
2. Current systems use a "store and forward" model where bedside wide-field digital fundus photography is obtained and then uploaded for remote grading by expert readers
3. Benefits: high sensitivity and specificity, objective documentation, being able to compare images longitudinally, sharing photos for outside consultations

References

1. Palmer EA, Flynn JT, Hardy RJ, *et al*. The Cryotherapy for retinopathy of prematurity cooperative group. Incidence and early course of retinopathy of prematurity. *Ophthalmol* 1991;98:1628–1640.

2. Good WV, Hardy RJ, Dobson V, *et al*. The incidence and course of retinopathy of prematurity: Findings from the early treatment for retinopathy of prematurity study. *Pediatrics* 2005;116:15–23.

3. Fierson WM, American Academy of Pediatrics Section on Ophthalmology, American Academy of Ophthalmology, American Association for Pediatric Ophthalmology and Strabismus, American Association of Certified Orthoptists. Screening examination of premature infants for retinopathy of prematurity. *Pediatrics* 2013;131:189–195.

4. Early treatment for retinopathy of prematurity cooperative G. Revised indications for the treatment of retinopathy of prematurity: Results of the early treatment for retinopathy of prematurity randomized trial. *Arch Ophthalmol* 2003;121:1684–1694.

5. White JE, Repka MX. Randomized comparison of diode laser photocoagulation versus cryotherapy for threshold retinopathy of prematurity: 3-year outcome. *J Pediatr Ophthalmol Strabismus* 1997;34:83–87.

6. Banach MJ, Ferrone PJ, Trese MT. A comparison of dense versus less dense diode laser photocoagulation patterns for threshold retinopathy of prematurity. *Ophthalmol* 2000;107:324–327.

7. Mintz-Hittner HA, Kennedy KA, Chuang AZ. BEAT-ROP Cooperative Group. Efficacy of intravitreal bevacizumab for stage 3+ retinopathy of prematurity. *N Engl J Med* 2011;364(7):603–615.

8. Lepore D, Quinn GE, Molle F, *et al*. Intravitreal bevacizumab versus laser treatment in type 1 retinopathy of prematurity: Report on fluorescein angiographic findings. *Ophthalmol* 2014.

9. Trese MT. Surgical therapy for stage V retinopathy of prematurity. A two-step approach. *Graefes Arch Clin Exp Ophthalmol* 1987;225(4):266–268.

10. Capone Jr, A, Trese MT. L*ens-sparing* vitreous surgery for tractional stage 4a retinopathy of prematurity retinal detachments. *Ophthalmol* 2001;108:2068–2070.

11. Prenner JL, Capone Jr, A, Trese MT. Visual outcomes after lens-sparing vitrectomy for stage 4A retinopathy of prematurity. *Ophthalmol* 2004;111:2271–2273.

12. Capone Jr, A, Trese MT. Stage 5 retinopathy of prematurity: Then and now. *Retina* 2006;26:721–723.

13. Photographic Screening for Retinopathy of Prematurity (Photo-ROP) Cooperative Group. The photographic screening for retinopathy of prematurity study (Photo-ROP). Primary outcomes. *Retina* 2008;28(3):S47–S54.

14. Chiang MF, Melia M, Buffenn AN, *et al*. Detection of clinically significant retinopathy of prematurity using wide-angle digital retinal photography: A report by the American Academy of Ophthalmology. *Ophthalmol* 2012;119(6):1272–1280.

SECTION 4:
HEREDITARY RETINAL
DEGENERATION

Chapter 15: Retinitis Pigmentosa

Sumeer Thinda and Ala Moshiri

1. Incidence of Retinitis Pigmentosa (RP)

a. 1 in 4,000

2. Inheritance Pattern of RP

a. AD, AR, X-linked.
   i. More than 50 genes identified including rhodopsin and RDS/peripherin.

3. Clinical Features

a. Typically bilateral and symmetric
b. Symptoms

   i. Nyctalopia
   ii. Decreased peripheral vision
   iii. Loss of visual acuity is late manifestation

c. Fundus findings

   i. Waxy optic nerve pallor
   ii. Arteriole narrowing
   iii. Bone spicule-like pigment changes
   iv. Posterior subcapsular cataract
   v. Vitreous cell may be present
   vi. Cystoid macular edema may be present

d. Phenotypic variations

　　i. RP sine pigmento

　　　　1. Absence of bone-spicules

　　ii. Unilateral RP

　　　　1. Important to follow as may have subclinical disease in the presumed uninvolved eye
　　　　2. May not be RP — see differential diagnosis

　　iii. Sectoral RP

　　　　1. 1 or 2 sectors of fundus involved
　　　　2. Sharp demarcation line between normal and abnormal retina
　　　　3. Symmetric
　　　　4. May be seen in X-linked RP carriers (females)

　　iv. Central RP

　　　　1. Macular involvement early in disease with progression from central peripheral retina

　　v. Pericentral RP

　　　　1. Ring scotoma within the central 20–30°

　　vi. Retinitis punctata albescens

　　　　1. Deep white retinal dots

　　vii. Leber congenital amaurosis

　　　　1. Infantile or early childhood form

4. Diagnostic Testing

a. Full-field electroretinogram (ERG)

　　i. Reduction in rod > cone function
　　ii. A-waves and b-waves both reduced
　　iii. Prolonged b-waves
　　iv. Extinguished ERG in late course of disease

b. Visual field (VF) testing or perimetry

　　i. Ring scotoma, central sparing
　　ii. kinetic VF testing preferred

c. Optical coherence tomography (OCT)

    i. Loss of outer retinal structures
    ii. Outer retinal tubulations
    iii. Inner retinal cystic changes

d. Fluorescein angiogram (FA)

    i. Diffuse mottled staining or window defects from retinal pigment epithelial and/or chorioretinal atrophy
    ii. Non-leaking cystoid macular edema

5. Clinical Course

a. Slowly progressive disease
b. Sectoral retinitis pigmentosa (RP) can be stationary or slowly progressive
c. Full-field ERG becomes extinguished later in disease course

6. Differential Diagnosis

a. Medications (Thioridazine)
b. Paraneoplastic syndromes: cancer associated/melanoma associated retinopathy (CAR/MAR)
c. Acute zonal occult outer retinopathy (AZOOR)
d. Old retinal vascular occlusion
e. Old retinal detachment
f. Trauma
g. Uveitis
h. Infections (Syphilis, diffuse unilateral subacute neuroretinitis (DUSN))
i. Retained metallic intraocular foreign body

7. Management

a. Posterior subcapsular cataract: may be a visually significant benefit from surgery in an earlier stage of RP
b. Cystoid macular edema

    i. Topical dorzolamide
    ii. Oral acetazolamide
    iii. Intravitreal triamcinolone

c. Nutritional supplements — may be beneficial in selected patients

    i. Vitamin A palmitate 15,000 IU/day
    ii. Decosahexaenoic acid (DHA) 200 mg/day
    iii. Lutein 12 mg/day
    iv. Avoid Vitamin E

d. Argus II pre-retinal implant for end stage disease
e. Sunglasses for UV light protection
f. Low vision referral
g. Follow-up every 1–2 years to look for treatable causes of vision loss and gauge rate of progression

8. Rule out Retinal Degenerations Associated With Systemic Treatable Disease

a. See Table 1 for list of systemic diseases associated with pigmentary retinopathy
b. Bassen–Kornzweig syndrome(Abetalipoproteinemia with deficiency of fat soluble vitamins — A, D, E, K)

    i. See Table 1 for ocular and systemic findings
    ii. Treatment

        a. Vitamin A supplementation 300 IU/kg/day
        b. Vitamin E supplementation 100 IU/kg/day
        c. Vitamin K supplementation 0.15 mg/kg/day for bleeding tendency
        d. Restrict dietary fat to improve steatorrhea

c. Friedreich-like Ataxia (with vitamin E deficiency)

    i. See Table 1 for ocular and systemic findings
    ii. Treatment

        1. Oral alpha-tocopheryl acetate 400–900 mg/day

d. Refsum's disease (with elevated phytanic acid levels)
    i. See Table 1 for ocular and systemic findings
    ii. Treatment

        1. Dietary restriction of phytanic acid, phytol and chlorophyll
        2. Supplementation with essential fatty acids and 100 IU/day vitamin E
        3. Plasmapheresis for severe metabolic disease

Table 1. Retinal Degenerations Associated with Systemic disease.

Disease	Inheritance Pattern	Ocular Findings	Systemic Findings
Alagille syndrome	AD	Posterior embryotoxon, pigmentary retinopathy	Bile duct paucity, intrahepatic cholestatic syndrome, cardiovascular abnormalities, vertebral defects, renal disease
Alstrom disease	AR	Pigmentary retinopathy	Obesity, hearing loss, DM, renal failure, heart failure
Bardet–Biedl syndrome	AR	Pigmentary retinopathy, can have macular involvement	Mild MR, polydactyly, obesity, hypogonadism, renal abnormalities
Bassen–Kornzweig syndrome (abetalipoproteinemia with deficiency of fat soluble vitamins)	AR	Pigmentary retinopathy	Spinocerebellar degeneration, peripheral neuropathy, steatorrhea, RBC show acanthocytosis, low serum lipid levels
Friedreich-likeataxia (with vitamin E deficiency)	AR	Pigmentary retinopathy	Ataxia, dysarthria, decreased deep tendon reflexes, decreased proprioception and vibratory sense
Kearns–Sayre syndrome	Mitochondrial	CPEO, pigmentary retinopathy	Heart block
Mucopolysaccharidoses			
Hunter syndrome	XR	Pigmentary retinopathy	Generally have course facial features, bone abnormalities, enlarged visceral organs, hearing loss, MR, cardiorespiratory disease
Hurler syndrome	AR	Pigmentary retinopathy, corneal clouding	
Sanfillipo syndrome	AR	Pigmentary retinopathy	

(Continued)

Table 1. (*Continued*)

Disease	Inheritance Pattern	Ocular Findings	Systemic Findings
Scheie syndrome	AR	Pigmentary retinopathy, corneal clouding	Each form also has its own unique findings
Myotonic dystrophy	AD	Christmas tree cataract, pigmentary retinopathy, pattern dystrophy, ciliary body detachment	Frontal balding, hypogonadism, muscle wasting, myotonia, cardiac abnormalities
Neonatal adrenoleukodystrophy	AR	Pigmentary retinopathy, optic atrophy, cataract, vitreous cell	Less severe form of Zellweger syndrome with no renal defects
Neuronal ceroid lipofuscinosis (Batten disease)	AR	Pigmentary retinopathy, may have bull's eye maculopathy	CNS deterioration with ataxia, seizures and dementia (age of onset and clinical course varies with subtype)
Olivopontocerebellar atrophy	AD	Pigmentary retinopathy, macular degeneration, external ophthalmoplegia	Spinocerebellar degeneration
Refsum disease	AR	Pigmentary retinopathy	Elevated phytanic acid levels, chronic polyneuropathy, hearing loss, cerebellar ataxia
Usher syndrome	AR	Pigmentary retinopathy	Congenital deafness

(*Continued*)

Table 1. (*Continued*)

Disease	Inheritance Pattern	Ocular Findings	Systemic Findings
Waardenburg syndrome	AD	Heterochromic iris, pigmentary retinopathy	Hearing loss, white forelock, dystopia canthorum
Zellweger syndrome (cerebrohepatorenal syndrome)	AR	Corneal edema, cataract, glaucoma, pigmentary retinopathy, optic atropy	Abnormal myelinogenesis and demyelination, hypotonia, hearing loss, cirrhosis, renal cysts

References

1. Hamel C. Retinitis pigmentosa. *Orphanet Journal of Rare Diseases* 2006;1:40.
2. Hartong DT, Berson EL, Dryja TP. Retinitis pigmentosa. *Lancet* 2006;368: 1795–1809.
3. Humayun MS, Dorn JD, da Cruz L, *et al.* Interim results from the international trial of Second Sight's visual prosthesis. *Ophthalmol* 2012;119:779–788.
4. Salvatore S, Fishman GA, Genead MA. Treatment of cystic macular lesions in hereditary retinal dystrophies. *Survey of Ophthalmology* 2013;58:560–584.
5. Michaelides M, Hardcastle AJ, Hunt DM, *et al.* Progressive cone and cone-rod dystrophies: phenotypes and underlying molecular genetic basis. *Survey of Ophthalmology* 2006;51:232–258.
6. Thiadens AA, Phan TM, Zekveld-Vroon RC, *et al.* Clinical course, genetic etiology, and visual outcome in cone and cone-rod dystrophy. *Ophthalmol* 2012;119:819–826.
7. Bhatti MT. Retinitis pigmentosa, pigmentary retinopathies, and neurologic diseases. *Current Neurology and Neuroscience Reports* 2006;6:403–413.
8. Grant CA, Berson EL. Treatable forms of retinitis pigmentosa associated with systemic neurological disorders. *International Ophthalmology Clinics* 2001;41:103–110.
9. Goldberg NR, Greenberg JP, Laud K, *et al.* Freund KB. Outer retinal tubulation in degenerative retinal disorders. *Retina* 2013;33:1871–1876.

Chapter 16:
Hereditary Chorioretinal Dystrophies

Sumeer Thinda and Ala Moshiri

Choroideremia

1. Incidence

a. 1 in 50,000

2. Inheritance Pattern

a. X-linked recessive
  i. CHM gene on chromosome 21 coding for RAB geranylgeranyl transferase escort protein.

3. Clinical Features

a. Childhood onset
b. Bilateral and symmetric
c. Symptoms

  i. Nyctalopia
  ii. Loss of peripheral vision
  iii. Loss of central visual acuity late in the disease
  iv. Can be asymptomatic (carriers)

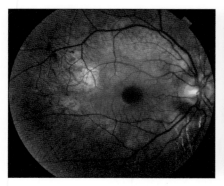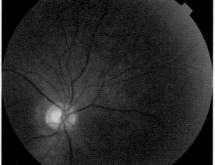

Figure 1. Fundus photograph of an eye with choroideremia (left) compared with that from the asymptomatic carrier mother (right). Note the mild peripheral pigment granularity of the carrier (Courtesy of Susanna S. Park, MD Phd).

d. Fundus findings (Figure 1)

  i. Atrophy of choroid and retinal pigment epithelium (RPE)
  ii. Normal retinal vessels and optic nerve (as opposed to findings in retinitis pigmentosa (RP))
  iii. Begins as RPE mottling which progresses to confluent scalloped areas of RPE and choriocapillaris loss
  iv. Larger choroidal vessels are preserved
  v. Carriers

    1. Patches of RPE mottling
    2. Lobular loss of RPE and choriocapillaris

4. Diagnostic Testing

a. Full-field electroretinogram (ERG)

  i. Rod > cone dysfunction
  ii. Extinguished late in disease
  iii. Normal in carriers

b. Visual Field

  i. Ring scotoma (kinetic perimetry testing preferred)

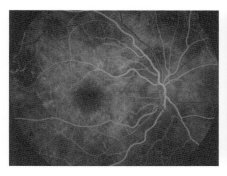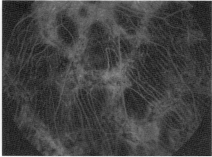

Figure 2. Fluorescein angiogram of choroideremia. Early transit view shows patches of window defect from chorioretinal degeneration. Mid transit view of periphery shows more prominent window defects through which large choroidal vessels are seen.

   c. Optical coherence tomography (OCT)

      i. Loss of outer retinal structures
     ii. Outer retinal tabulations
    iii. Inner retinal cystic changes
    iv. RPE degeneration

   d. Fluorescein Angiography (Figure 2)

      i. Areas of hypofluoresence (corresponding to absent choriocapillaris) adjacent to areas of hyperfluorescense (corresponding to preserved choriocapillaris)

5. Clinical Course

a. Slowly progressive diffuse degeneration of RPE and choriocapillaris.
b. Most have visual acuity worse than 20/200 by age 50

6. Differential Diagnosis

a. Medications (thioridazine)
b. Gyrate atrophy
c. Bietti crystalline dystrophy
d. RP

7. Management

a. Low vision referral
b. Follow-up annually

Gyrate Atrophy

1. Incidence

Highest incidence in Finland

2. Inheritance Pattern

a. AR

    i. Gene on chromosome 10 encoding OAT (ornithine aminotransferase)

3. Clinical Features

a. Childhood onset
b. Bilateral and symmetric
c. Symptoms

    i. Nyctalopia
    ii. Loss of peripheral vision
    iii. Loss of central visual acuity late in the disease

d. Fundus findings

    i. Starts as areas of peripheral paving stone-like atrophy of RPE and choroid which enlarge and coalesce with scalloped borders
    ii. Hyperpigmentation of remaining RPE (which helps to differentiate this condition from choroideremia)
    iii. Progressive myopia
    iv. Cataracts (posterior sutural)

4. Diagnostic Testing

a. Full-field ERG

    i. Rod > cone dysfunction
    ii. Extinguished late in disease

b. Visual Field

    i. Ring scotoma (kinetic perimetry testing preferred)

c. OCT

    i. Loss of outer retinal structures

    ii. Outer retinal tubulations

    iii. Inner retinal cystic changes

    iv. Hyperreflective deposits in ganglion cell layer

    v. RPE degeneration

d. Flourescein Angiography

    i. Areas of hypofluoresence (corresponding to absent choriocapillaris) adjacent to areas of hyperfluorescense (corresponding to preserved choriocapillaris

5. Clinical Course

a. Slowly progressive diffuse degeneration of RPE and choriocapillaris

b. Central vision typically preserved until 30 or 40 years of age

6. Differential Diagnosis

a. Medications (thioridazine)

b. Choroideremia

c. Bietti crystalline dystrophy

d. Retinitis pigmentosa

7. Diagnosis

a. Serum ornithine levels

b. Genetic analysis of OAT gene

8. Management

a. Dietary restriction of arginine

b. Vitamin B6 (pyridoxine)

c. Low vision referral

d. Follow-up every 6–12 months

References

1. Agarwal A. Gass' Atlas of Macular Diseases, 5th edn., Saunders, 2011.
2. Coussa RG, Traboulsi EI. Choroideremia: A review of general findings and pathogenesis. *Ophthalmic Genetics* 2012;33:57–65.
3. Syed R, Sundquist SM, Ratnam K, *et al.* High-resolution images of retinal structure in patients with choroideremia. *Investigative Ophthalmology & Visual Science* 2013;54:950–961.
4. Sergouniotis PI, Davidson AE, Lenassi E, *et al.* Retinal structure, function, and molecular pathologic features in gyrate atrophy. *Ophthalmol* 2012;119:596–605.

Chapter 17: Cone Dystrophy

Sumeer Thinda and Ala Moshiri

Cone Dystrophy

1. Incidence

a. 1 in 30,000 to 1 in 40,000

2. Inheritance Patterns

a. AD, AR, X linked
b. More than 10 genes identified

3. Clinical Features

a. Onset teenage years to adulthood
b. Bilateral and symmetric
c. Symptoms

    i. Loss of central visual acuity
    ii. Hemeralopia
    iii. Photophobia

d. Fundus findings

    i. Bull's eye pattern macular atrophy
    ii. Temporal optic nerve pallor

4. Diagnostic Testing

a. Full Field Electroretinography (ffERG)

    i. Reduction in cone function with normal or near normal rod function.

    ii. May have rod involvement later in disease (overlap with cone-rod dystrophy)

b. Visual Field

    i. Normal peripheral visual fields early in disease (may have peripheral visual field loss late in disease)

c. Optical coherence tomography (OCT)

    i. Loss of macular outer retinal structures

    ii. Outer retinal tubulations

d. Fluorescein Angiography

    i. Macular window defect corresponding to macular atrophy

5. Clinical Course

a. Progressive disease

b. May have rod dysfunction late in disease (overlap with cone-rod dystrophy)

6. Differential Diagnosis

a. Stargardt's disease

b. Central areolar choroidal dystrophy

c. North Carolina macular dystrophy

d. Olivopontocerebellar atrophy

e. Ceroid lipofuscinosis

f. Age related macular degeneration

g. Toxic maculopathy (chloroquine)

7. Management

a. Dark sunglasses or miotics for photophobia

b. Low vision referral

c. Follow-up every 1–2 years

References

1. Michaelides M, Hardcastle AJ, Hunt DM, *et al.* Progressive cone and cone-rod dystrophies: Phenotypes and underlying molecular genetic basis. *Survey of Ophthalmology* 2006;51:232–258.
2. Thiadens AA, Phan TM, Zekveld-Vroon RC, *et al.* Clinical course, genetic etiology, and visual outcome in cone and cone-rod dystrophy. *Ophthalmol* 2012;119:819–826.
3. Hamel CP. Cone rod dystrophies. *Orphanet Journal of Rare Diseases* 2007;2:7.

Chapter 18: Hereditary Maculopathy

Sumeer Thinda and Ala Moshiri

STARGARDT'S DISEASE

1. Incidence

a. 1 in 8,000 to 1 in 10,000
b. Most common hereditary macular dystrophy of childhood

2. Inheritance Pattern

a. Autosomal recessive (AR) (most common), autosomal dominant (AD)

    i. Multiple genes identified, most common is ABCA4 on chromosome 1

3. Clinical Features

a. Juvenile onset
b. Bilateral and symmetric
c. Symptoms

    i. Loss of central visual acuity
    ii. Hemeralopia
    iii. Photophobia

d. Fundus findings

    i. Bull's eye pattern macular atrophy
    ii. Pisciform flecks at the level of the retinal pigment epithelium (RPE)

4. Diagnostic Testing

a. Full-field electroretinogram (ERG)

    i. Reduction in cone function

ii. Can have variable rod involvement (overlap with cone-rod dystrophy)

b. Visual Field Test

    i. Can range from normal to constricted peripheral visual fields (kinetic perimetry testing preferred)

    ii. Central scotoma corresponding the degree of macular involvement

c. Optical coherence tomography (OCT)

    i. Loss of macular outer retinal structures

    ii. Outer retinal tubulations

d. Fundus autofluorescence (AF)

    i. Hyper or hypo-autofluoresence of pisciform flecks depending on age of fleck (new versus old atrophic fleck)

    ii. Hypo-autofluorescence within area of atrophy

e. Flourescein Angiography

    i. Dark (silent) choroid — See Fig. 1

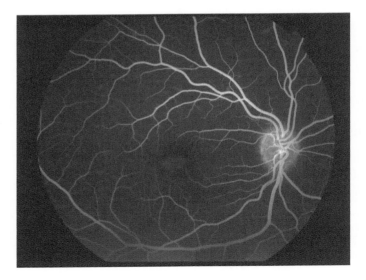

Figure 1. Fluorescein angiogram of Stagard't Disease. Mid-transit view showing the characteristic "dark choroid" resulting from diffuse blocked fluorescence from lipofuscin accumulation in the retinal pigment epithelium. A faint hyperfluorescence from an early window defect or staining is seen in the central macula from maculopathy. Some faint staining of the flecks are noted along the supratemporal arcade.

    ii. Pisciform flecks may be either hypofluorescent or hyperfluoresecent depending on age of fleck

    iii. Macular hyperfluorescent window defect corresponding to macular atrophy

5. Clinical Course

a. Slowly progressive

b. Most patients will have vision between 20/50 and 20/200

c. Can have peripheral degenerative changes with corresponding visual function (VF) and ERG loss

6. Differential Diagnosis

Same as cone dystrophy for Bull's eye maculopathy

a. Sunglasses for UV light protection

b. Low vision referral

c. Follow-up every 1–2 years

BEST'S DISEASE

1. Inheritance Pattern

a. AD

    i. BEST1 gene on chromosome 11 encoding bestrophin

2. Clinical Features

a. Childhood onset

b. Bilateral and symmetric

c. Symptoms

    i. Loss of central visual acuity

    ii. Metamorphosis

d. Fundus findings

    i. Stage 0: normal fundus exam

    ii. Stage 1: RPE mottling

    iii. Stage 2a: vitelliform macular lesion ("egg yolk appearance"), 30% can have extra-macular lesions

iv. Stage 2b: vitelliruptive macular lesion ("scrambled egg appearance")

v. Stage 3: pseudohypopyon macular lesion with development of fluid level

vi. Stage 4a: geographic atrophy

vii. Stage 4b: subretinal fibrosis

viii. Stage 4c: Choroidal neovascularization (CNVM)

3. Diagnostic Testing

a. Full-field ERG

    i. Normal

b. Electooculogram (EOG)

    i. Abnormal with Arden ratio typically <1.5

c. Visual Field Test

    i. Normal peripheral vision

d. OCT

    i. Depends on stage of disease

        1. Presence of subretinal vitelliform material early in the disease

        2. Areas of RPE atrophy and outer retinal loss later in the disease

        3. Pigment epithelial detachment, subretinal and interstitial fluid associated with CNVM in late stage

e. Fundus Autofluorescence

    i. Depends on stage of disease

        1. Hyperautofluoresence of vitelliform material

        2. Hypoautofluorescence of RPE atrophy later in the disease

f. Fluorescein Angiography

    i. Depends on stage of disease

        1. Early blockage with late staining of vitelliform material

        2. Window defect of geographic atrophy

        3. Staining of subretinal fibrosis

        4. Leakage from CNVM

4. Clinical Course

a. Slowly progressive
b. Most retain 20/40 or better unless develop CNVM
c. 20% develop CNVM

5. Differential Diagnosis

a. Pattern dystrophy (adult onset foveomacular vitelliform dystrophy)
b. Cuticular drusen with vitelliform material
c. Drusneoid RPE detachment
d. Stargardt's disease
e. Cone and cone-rod dystrophy
f. Central areolar choroidal dystrophy
g. Age related macular degeneration
h. Toxic maculopathy (chloroquine)

6. Management

a. Low vision referral
b. Follow-up every 6–12 months depending on stage

PATTERN DYSTROPHY

1. Inheritance Pattern

a. Typically AD

  i. Associated gene: RDS/peripherin

2. Clinical Features

a. Midlife onset
b. Unilateral or bilateral
c. Symptoms

  i. Decrease in central visual acuity
  ii. Metamorphosis
  iii. Can be asymptomatic (incidental finding)

d. Fundus findings (4 phenotypic variants)

  i. Adult onset foveomacular vitelliform dystrophy
    1. Yellow subfoveal lesion with central pigmented spot

2. Typically 1/3 Disc diameter in size
ii. Butterfly dystrophy
   1. Butterfly like pattern of yellow or brown pigment clumping
iii. Reticular dystrophy
   1. Fishnet like pattern of yellow or brown pigment clumping
iv. Fundus pulverulentus
   1. Course pigment clumping
v. Clinical phenotype can vary between the 2 eyes and the subtype can evolve from one to another in the same eye

3. Diagnostic Testing

a. Full-field ERG

  i. Normal

b. EOG

  i. Borderline or mildly reduced

c. Visual Field Test

  i. Normal peripheral vision

d. OCT

  i. Depends on phenotypic variant:

    1. Subretinal vitelliform material
    2. Dome shaped elevations in RPE corresponding to RPE clumping

e. Fluorescein Angiography

  i. Areas of central hypofluorescence with surrounding hyperfluoresence

4. Clinical Course

a. May develop geographic atrophy
b. Small risk of CNVM development

5. Differential Diagnosis

a. Age related macular degeneration
b. Chronic central serous chorioretinopathy
c. Drusenoid RPE detachment
d. Best's disease

6. Management

a. Follow-up annually

CENTRAL AREOLAR CHOROIDAL DYSTROPHY

1. Inheritance Pattern

a. AD, most common and AR

2. Clinical Features

a. Midlife onset
b. Bilateral and symmetric
c. Symptoms
d. Loss of central visual acuity
e. Fundus findings

    i. Early macular RPE mottling with later development of geographic atrophy

    ii. Can have drusen-like changes

f. Full-field ERG

    i. Normal

    ii. May have cone dysfunction in advanced disease

g. Visual Field Test

    i. Normal peripheral vision

h. OCT

    i. Loss of outer retinal structures

    ii. RPE degeneration

i. Fluorescein angiogram

    i. Window defect from area of macular atrophy

3. Clinical Course

a. Slowly progressive
b. Loss of Visual acuity occurs between 30 and 60 years of age

4. Differential Diagnosis

Same as cone dystrophy

5. Management

a. Low vision referral
b. Follow-up annually

NORTH CAROLINA MACULAR DYSTROPHY

1. Inheritance Pattern

a. AD

2. Clinical Features

a. Infancy onset
b. Bilateral and symmetric
c. Symptoms

   i. Metamorphopsia
   ii. Loss of central visual acuity

d. Fundus findings (3 phenotypic grades)

   i. Grade 1: yellow or white peculiar drusen-like deposits
   ii. Grade 2: confluent drusen, RPE changes, geographic atrophy, subretinal fibrosis
   iii. Grade 3: macular staphyloma or caldera

3. Diagnositic Testing

a. Full-field ERG

   i. Normal

b. Visual Field Test

   i. Normal peripheral vision

c. OCT

    i. Depends on phenotypic grade

        1. Loss of outer retinal structures
        2. RPE degeneration
        3. Staphyloma or caldera
        4. Intrachoroidal cavitations

d. Fluorescein Angiography

    i. Window defect from area of macular atrophy
    ii. Straining of subretinal fibrosis
    iii. Leakage of CNVM

4. Clinical Course

a. Macular changes tend to stabilize by the teenage years
b. Vision ranges from 20/20 to 20/200
c. Can rarely develop CNVM

5. Differential Diagnosis

Same as cone dystrophy

a. Stargardt's disease
b. Central areolar choroidal dystrophy
c. North Carolina macular dystrophy
d. Olivopontocerebellar atrophy
e. Ceroid lipofuscinosis
f. Age related macular degeneration
g. Toxic maculopathy (chloroquine)

6. Management

a. Low vision referral
b. Follow-up every 6–12 months depending on phenotypic grade

References

1. Armstrong JD, Meyer D, Xu S, *et al.* Long-term follow-up of Stargardt's disease and fundus flavimaculatus. *Ophthalmol* 1998;105:448–457.
2. Walia S, Fishman GA. Natural history of phenotypic changes in Stargardt macular dystrophy. *Ophthalmic Genetics* 2009;30:63–68.
3. MacDonald IM, Lee T. Best vitelliform macular dystrophy. *GeneReviews*. Seattle, WA: University of Washington, Seattle, 2013.
4. Agarwal A. Gass' Atlas of Macular Diseases, Fifth Edition. Saunders, 2011.
5. Coon CJ, Klevering BJ, Cremers FP, *et al.* Central areolar choroidal dystrophy. *Ophthalmol* 2009;116:771–782.
6. Schoenberger SD, Agarwal A. Intrachoroidal cavitation in North Carolina macular dystrophy. *JAMA ophthalmol* 2013;131:1073–1076.
7. Khurana RN, Sun X, Pearson E, *et al.* A reappraisal of the clinical spectrum of North Carolina macular dystrophy. *Ophthalmol* 2009;116:1976–1983.
8. Goldberg NR, Greenberg JP, Laud K, *et al.* Outer retinal tubulation in degenerative retinal disorders. *Retina* 2013;33:1871–1876.

SECTION 5:
POSTERIOR UVEITIS

Chapter 19: Work Up and Management of Uveitis

Elad Moisseiev and Susanna S. Park

1. Nomenclature of Uveitis

The Standardization of Uveitis Nomenclature (SUN) workgroup has developed an internationally accepted scheme for classifying uveitis. The following definitions are of clinical importance:

A. *Anatomic location* — the primary site of ocular inflammation serves as the framework for diagnosing uveitis

- Anterior uveitis — primarily in the anterior chamber, including iritis, iridocyclitis and anterior cyclitis
- Intermediate uveitis — primarily in the vitreous, including posterior cyclitis, pars planitis and vitritis
- Posterior uveitis — primarily in the retina or choroid, including retinitis, retinochoroiditis, chorioretinitis and choroiditis
- Panuveitis — when there is no predominant site, and inflammation involves the anterior chamber, vitreous and retina and/or choroid
- It should be remembered that presence of peripheral vascular sheathing, neovascularization or CME does not change the classification

B. *Timing descriptors* — episodes of uveitis may be temporally defined

- Onset — sudden or insidious
- Duration — limited (under 3 months) or persistent (over 3 months)

- Course — is classified as:
    - Acute — an episode of sudden onset and limited duration
    - Recurrent — repeated episodes separated by periods of inactivity without treatment over 3 months in duration
    - Chronic — persistence of uveitis with relapse in less than 3 months after stopping treatment

C. *Grading of inflammatory ocular findings*

- The following standardized grading scales for anterior chamber cells, anterior chamber flare and vitreous haze are used clinically:

Table 1.

Grade	Anterior Chamber Cells	Anterior Chamber Flare	Vitreous Haze
0	<1 cells in field	none	none
0.5+	1–5 cells in field	—	minimal (posterior pole clearly visible)
1+	6–15 cells in field	faint	mild (posterior pole details slightly hazy)
2+	16–25 cells in field	moderate (iris and lens details clear)	moderate (posterior pole details very hazy)
3+	26–50 cells in field	marked (iris and lens details hazy)	marked (posterior pole details barely visible)
4+	>50 cells in field	intense (presence of fibrin or plastic aqueous)	severe (posterior pole not visible)

- No scales for grading hypopyon, vitreous cells or keratic precipitates exist

D. *Response descriptors* — responses to treatment of uveitis are defined as:

- Inactive — grade 0 cells
- Worsening activity — a two-step increase in inflammation or increase from grade 3+ to 4+
- Improved activity — a two-step decrease in inflammation or decrease to grade 0
- Remission—inactive disease over 3 months after stopping treatment

E. *Additional definitions of clinical importance*

- Uveitic glaucoma — elevated intraocular pressure in the presence of uveitis should not be considered as glaucoma and this term is reserved for cases with documented glaucomatous optic disc damage or visual field defect
- Trace (or 0.5+) cells still indicated disease activity and cannot be considered as inactive
- Successful corticosteroid sparing — is considered when the dose of prednisone is reduced to 10 mg/day or less (or its equivalent for other corticosteroids)
- Pars planitis — reserved for cases with intermediate uveitis in the absence of an infection or systemic disease (idiopathic)

2. Epidemiology of Uveitis

- The incidence, prevalence and distribution of uveitis vary between different geographic locations and ethnic backgrounds
- Overall, uveitis is responsible for 2.8–10% of all cases of blindness
- Worldwide incidence is estimated at 17–52 per 100,000 in the population per year; prevalence is estimated at 38–714 cases per 100,000 in the population
- Anterior uveitis is the most common type, accounting for over half of the cases in the western world. Posterior uveitis is the second most common type, accounting for 15–30% of cases. This is followed by panuveitis and intermediate uveitis is the least common type
- Most cases of uveitis present between the ages of 20–60 years
- In children, posterior uveitis is more common than anterior uveitis (most common reasons for posterior uveitis in children are toxoplasmosis and idiopathic and JIA (juvenile idiopathic arthritis) for anterior uveitis)
- Masquerade syndromes, most notably ocular lymphoma (primary or part of CNS lymphoma), should be considered in the differential diagnosis, especially in elderly patients

3. Initial Evaluation

A. *History* — thorough history taking is often very important in diagnosing uveitis. The following issues should be addressed:

- Medical history — background systemic diseases, medications, surgeries

- Additional signs and symptoms — such as fever, fatigue, weight loss, night sweats, headaches, hearing loss, tinnitus, rashes, aphthous lesions, genital sores, hair loss or discoloration, cough, diarrhea, back and joint pain or stiffness and bloody urine
- Ocular history — previous ocular diseases or surgeries, previous episodes of uveitis
- History of travel, exposure to animals, insect bites or consumption of raw meats or other non-processed foods, drinking from stream or wells
- History should also include allergies, pregnancy, smoking, alcohol consumption, drug use
- Family history — of systemic and ocular diseases, including uveitis

B. *Physical examination* — a complete ophthalmic examination of both eyes should always be performed, and often a general physical examination is also in order

C. *Diagnosis* — based on the history and findings on examination, the uveitis can be classified and a differential diagnosis can be made. Further diagnostic tests should be ordered after a differential has been established. Infectious etiologies and systemic autoimmune causes need to be ruled out since treatment and management will vary. Occult malignancy masquarading as uveitis should also be considered in select cases

4. Anterior Uveitis

A. *Epidemiology*

- The most common type of uveitis, accounting for 50–75% of all cases
- Less common in Asian populations

B. *Differential diagnosis*

1. Idiopathic

   - The majority of cases are idiopathic (over 50%), with negative work-up
   - Some advocate not performing any work-up upon the initial presentation, unless additional ocular or systemic signs of involvement are present, but only in cases of recurrence

2. HLA–B27 associated uveitis

   - HLA–B27 is positive in over 50% of Caucasians presenting with acute anterior uveitis, while its frequency in the general population is 8%

- More common in young adult males
- Entities associated with HLA–B27 include ankylosing spondylitis, Reiter's syndrome, psoriasis, inflammatory bowel disease and some JIA
- History should include back pain or stiffness and a sacroiliac joint X-ray may be considered

3. Fuch's heterochromic iridocyclitis

   - Typically unilateral but may be bilateral in up to 15% of cases
   - Occurs commonly in young adults
   - Examination is often positive for typical diffuse, small stellate-shaped keratic precipitates. Abnormal vessels crossing the angle may often be seen by gonioscopy
   - Often associated with early progression of cataract, glaucoma and CME

4. Glaucomatous cyclitic crisis (Posner–Schlossman syndrome)

   - Recurrent episodes of anterior uveitis and elevated IOP
   - More common in older patients

5. Tubulointerstitial nephritis and uveitis (TINU)

   - Typically occurs in young females, often under 20
   - Cellular casts consistent with nephritis are found in urine

6. Juvenile idiopathic arthritis (JIA)

   - The most common cause of anterior uveitis in children
   - Routine ophthalmic examinations are required since uveitis may be asymptomatic and diagnosed at a late stage
   - Typical patients are young girls with pauciarticular JIA, with positive ANA

7. Infectious causes — common pathogens to rule out include herpes simplex virus (HSV), herpes zoster virus (HZV), syphilis, TB, lyme and toxoplasmosis

5. Intermediate Uveitis

A. *Epidemiology*

- The least common type of uveitis

B. *Differential diagnosis*

1. Pars planitis

   - The most common form of intermediate uveitis
   - Cases must be idiopathic
   - Typically occurs in young adults
   - Corticosteroids are the mainstay of treatment

2. Other causes of intermediate uveitis

   - Multiple sclerosis (MS) — 1–2.5% of MS patients may have intermediate uveitis. Up to 15% of patients with pars planitis may eventually be diagnosed with MS
   - Lyme disease
   - HTLV–1 associated uveitis

6. Posterior Uveitis

A. *Epidemiology*

   - The second most common type of uveitis

B. *Differential diagnosis*

1. Infectious causes

   - The most common cause worldwide, due to high prevalence of toxoplasmosis, TB and onchocerciasis in the developing world. Other possible causes include viral, lyme, syphilis, bartonella and fungal

2. Collagen vascular diseases

   - May cause posterior uveitis and retinal vasculitis
   - Depending on whether arteries or veins are affected, different etiologies should be considered:
     o Predominantly Retinal Periphlebitis:
       ▪ Perivenous sheathing, retinal vein occlusion and exudation
       ▪ e.g. Multiple Sclerosis or Sarcoidosis
     o Predominantly Retinal Arteritis:
       ▪ Cotton wool spots, retinal artery occlusion
       ▪ e.g. Systemic lupus erythematosus (SLE), Scleroderma, Giant cell arteritis and polyarteritis nodosa

o Combined Retinal Arteritis and Periphlebitis:

  ▪ e.g. Behcets and Wegener's granulomatosis

3. Presumed ocular histoplasmosis syndrome (POHS)

   • Almost exclusively found in the Ohio–Mississippi valley, where positive reactivity to histoplasmin skin test is very common.
   • Classical clinical triad includes multiple white, atrophic choroidal scars (histo-spots), peripapillary pigment changes, and choroidal neovascularization. No vitritis is present

4. White-dot syndromes

   • A heterogeneous group of auto-immune inflammatory chorioretinopathies, characterized by the presence of multiple white or yellow lesions at the level of the outer retina, RPE or choroid
   • The following is a summary of the important clinical characteristics of white dot syndromes:

Entity	Gender	Laterality	Findings	Important Characteristics
APMPPE (acute posterior multifocal placoid pigment epitheliopathy)	M = F	Bi	Multifocal, flat, creamy white or grayish placoid lesions at RPE level about 1 disc area or smaller in size in posterior pole. Typically resolve within few weeks with marked pigment alteration. (Figure 1)	Young, healthy adults; Associated with viral prodrome. Good prognosis for almost full recovery of vision with observation. Atypical cases may be complicated by CNS vasculitis or panuveitis requiring systemic corticosteroid therapy

(Continued)

(*Continued*)

Serpiginous choroiditis	M > F	Bi — asymmetric		Grey creamy choroidal lesions starting around the disc and macula leading to geographic pattern of RPE atrophy, centripetal expansion from recurrent activity at border of scars	Middle-aged adults; May cause choroidal neovascularization (CNV) macular edema or scarring; mild vitritis may be present
MEWDS (multiple evanescent white dot syndrome)	F > M	80% Uni		Small faint, transient white dots at level of outer retina and RPE. Mild transient vitritis and disc edema	Young healthy females usually. associated with viral prodrome. Blind spot enlargement may be present and persist. Good prognosis with observation
Birdshot chorioretinopathy	F > M	Bi		Multiple ovoid small vitiliginous lesions. Typically nasal to disc and along vessels, radiating peripherally. Vitritis correlates with acitivity (Figure 2)	Middle-aged; >90% are HLA-A29 positive May cause cystoid macular edema or CNV which limit vision

(*Continued*)

(Continued)

MCP (multifocal choroiditis with panuveitis)	F > M	80% Bi	Yellow-gray choroidal lesions that are later replaced by "punched-out" lesions	Myopic young healthy women; Can differentiate from POHS by presence of vitritis which often recur; May cause CME and CNV Poor prognosis
PIC (punctate inner choroiditis)	F > M	Bi	Discrete, well circumscribed white-yellow lesions <300 um size confined to the macula leading to scarring (Figure 3)	Myopic young healthy women; No vitritis. Paracentral or central scotoma acutely; May cause CNV with resolution limiting vision
AZOOR (acute zonal occult outer retinopathy)	F > M	Bi	Areas of RPE atrophy and pigmentary changes with corresponding perimetry defect and ERG abnormality	Can occur after MEWS or MCP; 30% have a systemic autoimmune disease May include perivascular sheathing

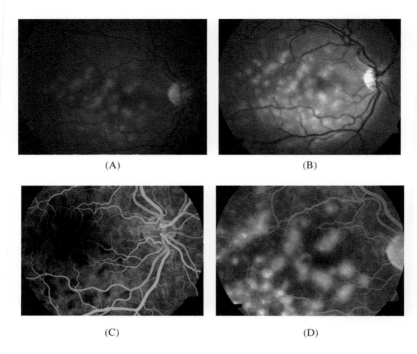

(A)   (B)

(C)   (D)

Figure 1. APMPPE, acute presentation: (A) Fundus photograph of the right eye at presentation of a 25 year old female patient with acute posterior multifocal placoid pigment epitheliopathy (APMPPE). (B) Infra-red image shows more vividly the multiple flat, whitish placoid lesions, about 1 disc area or smaller, in the posterior pole. (C) Fluorescent angiography early transit demonstrates early hypofluorescence. (D) Late transit fluorescein angiogram shows the classic late hyperfluorescence of the lesions. Findings were similar bilaterally.

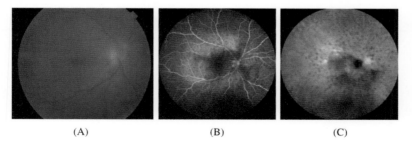

(A)   (B)   (C)

Figure 2. Birdshot Choroiditis: (A) The fundus photograph of the right eye of a 57 year old man with Birdshot chorioretinopathy, who presented with mild optic disc swelling and vitritis. (B) Fluorescein angiogram showing some blocked fluorescence from vitreous opacity. (C) Indocyanine green angiogram demonstrates multifocal spots of hypofluorescence radiating out to the periphery characteristic of this condition.

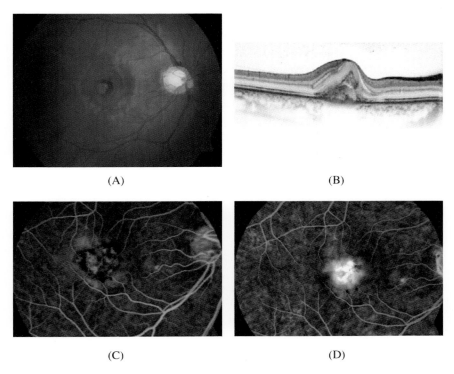

(A) (B)

(C) (D)

Figure 3. Punctate Inner Choroiditis (PIC): Right eye of a 30 year old female patient with a history of PIC. (A) Color fundus photograph showing a subfoveal gray elevated lesion from scarring. (B) OCT line scan demonstrates focal loss of photoreceptors and disruption of the retinal architecture at the foveal. Subretinal lesion suggestive of fibrosis is seen. (C) Fluorescein angiography early transit demonstrates early hypofluorescence with a rim of hypo fluorescence. (D) Late transit angiogram showing hyperfluorescence from staining of the macular lesion.

7. Panuveitis

A. *Epidemiology*

- The third most common type of uveitis

B. *Differential diagnosis*

1. Sarcoidosis

   - A systemic granulomatous inflammatory disease that can involve any organ in the body (most common — lung, lymph nodes, skin). Approximately half of patients will have ocular involvement

- More common in African-American patients
- Ocular sarcoidosis can affect any part of the eye. Common manifestations include anterior uveitis in as many as 60% of patients. Classic signs include large ("mutton-fat") keratic precipitates (KPs), iritis and iris nodules. Up to a third of patients have posterior uveitis, whose classic signs include dense vitritis and perivenous sheathing ("candle-wax dripping"). Rarer manifestations include optic neuropathy, subretinal neovascularization and choroidal granulomas
- Definitive diagnosis requires biopsy. Often the diagnosis is made based on clinical suspicion and chest CT or X-ray, Pulmonary function tests (PFTs), Gallium scan and elevated serum ACE or lysozyme levels
- Treatment is often systemic corticosteroids and in cases requiring prolonged treatment steroid-sparing immunomodulatory drugs are used

2. Behcet disease

    - A systemic disease, characterized by the classic triad of recurrent aphthous ulcers in the oral mucosa, skin and genital ulcers and uveitis
    - Diagnosis is based on clinical suspicion (there are criteria established by the International Study Group for Behcet Disease)
    - More common in the Mediterranean basin and Far East
    - The disease is associated with HLA-B51.
    - Ocular involvement is usually bilateral and often "explosive". Manifestations include iridocyclitis, with hypopion formation in about a third of cases (which typically shifts when head is tilted), posterior synechiae, retinal vascular occlusions, retinal hemorrhages and edema and marked vitritis. Rarer manifestations include episcleritis, keratitis and extraocular muscle paralysis
    - Treatment often starts with systemic corticosteroids, but most patients require prolonged treatment or become resistant and require immunomodulatory agents

3. Vogt–Koyanagi–Harada (VKH) syndrome

    - A systemic disorder, presumed to occur due to erroneous autoimmune sensitization of T lymphocytes against melanocytes

- VKH is diagnosed clinically based on the following criteria:

    i. No history of ocular trauma or surgery
    ii. No clinical or lab evidence of other ocular or systemic disease
    iii. Bilateral ocular disease, with either:

    Early manifestations — diffuse choroiditis with subretinal fluid or exudative retinal detachment and typical multiple pinpoint leaks on FA
    Late manifestations — ocular depigmentation, RPE clumping, recurrent anterior uveitis

    iv. Neurologic and auditory findings — meningismus, tinnitus, CSF pleocytosis.
    v. Integumentary findings — alopecia, poliosis, vitiligo

    * i–iii = probable; i–iii + iv/v = incomplete; i–v = complete

- FA has a typical pattern of multiple pinpoint areas of leakage at the level of RPE, which later coalesce. There is also hyperfluorescent staining of the optic disc
- Ocular involvement is usually bilateral and typically has the following course:

    i. Prodrome phase — no ocular involvement. Headache with neck stiffness, neurological and auditory findings may be present; typically about 2 weeks prior to uveitis
    ii. Acute uveitic phase — blurred vision, granulomatous anterior uveitis, vitritis, exudative retinal detachment
    iii. Convalescent phase — resolution of retinal detachment with choroidal depigmentation, limbal depigmentation, vitiligo, poliosis, alopecia
    iv. Chronic phase — episodes of recurrent anterior uveitis can occur in 50% of cases.

- Systemic corticosteroids are the mainstay of treatment for VKH

4. Sympathetic ophthalmia (SO)

- Bilateral, diffuse granulomatous inflammation that occurs following surgical or accidental trauma to one eye (the exciting eye), that involves the other uninjured eye (sympathizing eye) after a latent period.

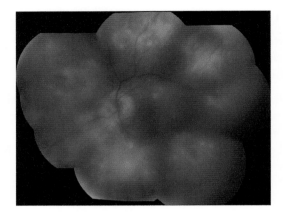

Figure 4.   Sympathetic Ophthalmia: This fundus photograph montage of the left eye of a 73 year old woman who had multiple retinal surgeries in her contralateral right eye showing vitreous opacity from vitritis, multifocal diffuse exudative retinal detachment and multiple choroidal granulomatous lesions (Dalen–Fuchs nodules) characteristic of sympathetic ophthalmia.

> Incarcerated uveal tissue may lead to autoimmune antibodies against ocular antigens
> - Inflammation may be more severe in the exciting eye
> - Typical ocular manifestations include mutton-fat KPs, iritis, posterior synechiae, vitritis, and choroidal granulomatous lesions (Dalen–Fuchs nodules, Figure 4). Additional manifestations include cataract, cystoid macular edema, CNV and optic atrophy
> - Ocular presentation is very similar to that of VKH — the key difference is lack of choriocapillaris involvement by SO
> - Enucleation of severely traumatized eye with no visual potential within 14 days of injury is recommended in order to prevent SO
> - Patients with treated with corticosteroids and also other immunosuppresants can maintain useful vision

8. Differential Diagnosis of Posterior and Panuveitis — in a Nutshell

- The following is a suggested differential diagnosis for posterior and panuveitis, based on the number of chorioretinal inflammatory foci and presence of vitritis:

Solitary Focal Chorioretinal Lesion		Multipolar Chorioretinal Lesions	
With Vitritis	Without Vitritis	With Vitritis	Without Vitritis
Toxoplasma	Neoplasia	Birdshot	POHS
Toxocara	Serpiginous	MCP	PIC
Sarcoidosis	TB	VKH	Serpiginous
TB	Sarcoidosis	Sympathetic	APMPPE
Cat-scratch		Ophthalmia	
		Sarcoidosis	
		Cat scratch	
		Viral Retinis	

9. Treatment of Uveitis

A. *General considerations*

- Choice of treatment agent, dosage and route of administration is made according to the specific diagnosis and etiology
- When uveitis is part of a systemic disease, treatment for control of the underlying systemic disease may be necessary
- When uveitis is complicated by elevated intraocular pressure, anti-glaucoma medications are used. Prostaglandin analogues should be used cautiously as they can exacerbate uveitis and CME

B. *Corticosteroids*

- Are the most commonly used agents for the acute treatment of uveitis. May be given topically, by periocular (subtenon) injection, by intravitreal injection, or systemically
- Ozurdex, a biodegradable slow release dexamethasone intravitreal implant, which is approved by the FDA for the treatment of non-infectious intermediate or posterior uveitis
- Long term treatment with topical steroids is associated with a multitude of adverse effects. Therefore, patients requiring prolonged treatment for disease control are often switched to immunomodulatory agents

C. *Immunomodulatory agents*

- The following diseases usually require such steroid-sparing long-term treatment: VKH, Behcet, sarcoidosis, serpiginous choroiditis, sympathetic ophthalmia, Birdshot, Wegener's, polyarteritis nodosa, JIA and necrotizing scleritis
- Classes of immunomodulatory agents:

Class	Examples of Agents	Mechanism of Action	Main Adverse Effects
Antimetabolites	Methotrexate, Azathioprine, Mycophenolate mofetil	Interfere with purine metabolism	GI upset, hepatotoxicity
T cell signaling inhibitors	Cyclosporine, Tacrolimus	Inhibit cytokines that activate lymphocytes	Nephrotoxicity, hypertension, GI upset
Alkylators	Cyclophosphamide, Chlorambucil	Cross-linking of DNA	Hemorrhagic cystitis, increased risk of malignancy
Biologic response modifiers	Infliximab	TNFα inhibitor	SLE-like autoimmune disease

10. Surgical Interventions in Uveitis

A. Surgery for the management of uveitis may be required for diagnostic or therapeutic reasons.

- Diagnostic procedures — aqueous tap, vitreous biopsy (vitreous tap or vitrectomy), tissue biopsy (from iris or choroid)
- Visual rehabilitation procedures — cataract extraction, removal of band keratopathy, synechiolysis and pupillary membrane removal, vitrectomy to remove dense vitrousopacities and membranes and epiretinal membrane peeling, Retisert implantation
- Procedures for the management of complications — glaucoma surgery, vitrectomy for clearing of vitreous hemorrhage, repair of retinal detachment or hypotony

B. Special considerations in surgery in uveitis

- Cataract extraction is non-urgent and is usually performed after 3 months of quiescence
- Cataract extraction surgery in uveitic eyes is complicated and associated with higher risk of postoperative complications, including hyphema, CME, glaucoma, postoperative inflammation and uveitis flare-up and posterior capsular opacification
- Glaucoma in eyes with uveitis may be due to reduced trabecular filtration secondary to anterior segment inflammation, posterior synechiae causing

pupillary block, anterior synechiae causing secondary angle closure, or in response to steroid treatment

- The preferred surgical technique for uveitic glaucoma is drainage device implantation (such as the Baerveldt or Ahmed valves)
- Indications for diagnostic vitrectomy include — atypical clinical presentations, non-response to treatment, rapidly progressive disease, or a suspicion for malignancy
- Vitrectomy in uveitic eyes is associated with higher risk of postoperative complications, including retinal detachment, vitreous hemorrhage and hypotony

References

1. Foster CS, Vitale AT. Diagnosis and treatment of uveitis. WB Saunders Company, 2002.
2. Nussenblatt RB, Whitcup SM, Palestine AG. Uveitis fundamentals and clinical practice. Mosby, 1996.
3. Basic and Clinical Science Course, Section 9: Intraocular inflammation and uveitis. *Am Acad Ophthalmol*, 2012–2013.
4. Jabs DA, Nussenblatt RB, Rosenbaum JT. Standardization of Uveitis Nomenclature (SUN) Working Group. Standardization of uveitis nomenclature for reporting clinical data. Results of the First International Workshop. *Am J Ophthalmol* 2005;140: 509–516.
5. Miserocchi E, Fogliato G, Modorati G *et al*. Review on the worldwide epidemiology of uveitis. *Eur J Ophthalmol* 2013;23:705–717.
6. Quillen DA, Davis JB, Gottlieb JL *et al*. The white dot syndromes. *Am J Ophthalmol* 2004;137:538–550.
7. Crawford CM1, Igboeli O. A review of the inflammatory chorioretinopathies: The white dot syndromes. *ISRN Inflamm* 2013;31:783190.
8. Lin P, Suhler EB, Rosenbaum JT. The future of uveitis treatment. *Ophthalmol* 2014; 121:365–376.
9. Lowder C, Belfort R Jr, Lightman S, *et al*. Ozurdex HURON Study Group. Dexamethasone intravitreal implant for non-infectious intermediate or posterior uveitis. *Arch Ophthalmol* 2011;129:545–553.
10. Murthy SI, Pappuru RR, Latha KM *et al*. Surgical management in patient with uveitis. *Indian J Ophthalmol* 2013;61:284–290.

Chapter 20: Infectious Uveitis

Senad Osmanovic and Susanna S. Park

Toxoplasmosis

1. Pathophysiology/Incidence

   a. Retinochoroiditis caused by protozoan parasite *Toxoplasma gondii*, specifically the tachyzoite stage

   b. Most common cause of posterior uveitis in the world

   c. May be congenital or acquired. Congenital infection is usually manifested within the first 4 years of life

   d. 2% of infected individuals from acquired toxoplasmosis may develop ocular manifestations

2. Clinical features (Figures 1 and 2)

   a. Focal area of white retinitis that is partially obscured by overlying vitritis, giving a "headlight in fog" appearance

   b. Old chorioretinal scars from previous activation may be present

   c. Kyrieleis plaques: Inflammatory plaques overlying arteries

   d. Presentation typically unilateral with single focus; bilateral disease and multifocality or diffuse inflammation should raise suspicion for immunocompromise

   e. Focal inflammation may result in branch arterial/venous occlusion

   f. Atypical presentations include punctate outer retinal toxoplasmosis (PORT): multifocal small white lesions in deep retina without vitritis

   g. Mild granulomatous anterior uveitis is typically seen

   h. Choroidal neovascularization can form in areas of old chorioretinal scarring

   i. Congenital infection may be accompanied by hydrocephalus and intracranial calcifications

3. Differential Diagnosis

    a. Toxocara granuloma
    b. Acute Retinal Necrosis
    c. Tuberculosis
    d. Syphilitic retinochoroiditis

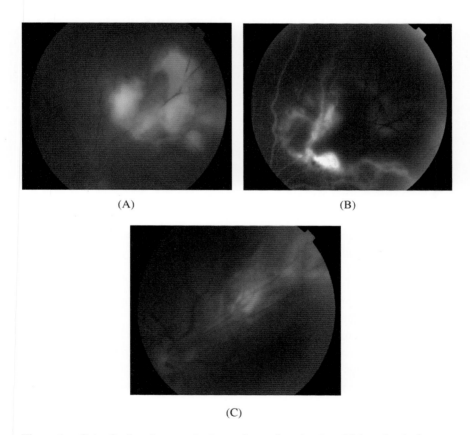

(A)   (B)

(C)

Figure 1. Color fundus photograph of toxoplasmosis retinochoroiditis and retinal vasculitis in a patient with AIDS showing exptensive retinitis without adjacent old scar (A). Fluorescein angiogram demonstrates extensive retinal ischemia peripheral to the retinitis due to retinal vascular occlusion from the associated retinal vasculitis (B). Following systemic therapy, the retinitis is completely resolved leaving a large area of scarring within the retina (C).

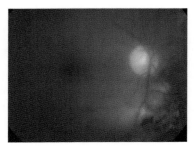

Figure 2. Fundus photograph of recurrent toxoplasma retinochoroiditis. New inflammatory lesion is typically seen at the periphery of an old chorioretinal scar in an immunocompetent patient. Diffuse vitritis is centered over the active inflammatory retinal lesion.

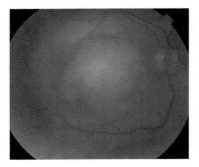

Figure 3. Fundus photography of placoid syphilitic chorioretinits in male patient with HIV. *Note*: Ill-defined deep yellow macular plaque with slight clearing in center.

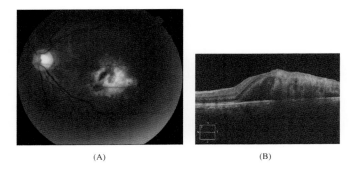

(A)   (B)

Figure 4. CMV retinitis involving the macula. (A) Fundus photograph of the macula showing the characteristic hemorrhagic retinitis with minimal vitritis in this patient with leukemia on chemotherapy awaiting bone marrow transplantation. (B) B-scan OCT image through the macula showing intraretinal infiltration.

4. Diagnostic testing

   a. Usually a clinical diagnosis based on above mentioned classic features
   b. Serum IgG may be obtained to confirm presence of exposure, but specificity is low since 30% of Americans are seropositive
   c. Negative serology effectively rules out *Toxoplasma* infection. IgM positivity indicates more recent exposure and may indicate primary retinochoroiditis
   d. *Goldmann–Witmer coefficient*: ratio of anti-toxoplasma IgG in aqueous to IgG in Serum. A value of 2 or above is indicative of intraocular involvement. This is rarely used in U.S.
   e. PCR of vitreous aspirate. It is more likely to be positive in primary infection versus recurrence/reactivation. May be utilized if antibody testing negative or inconclusive but clinical presentation is suggestive of toxoplasma. Aqueous aspirate has lower sensitivity due to poor penetration of organisms into the anterior chamber

5. Treatment

   a. Decision to initiate treatment is specific to lesion location and host factors. Small peripheral lesions in immunocompetent patients may be closely observed
   b. Treatment indicated for:

      i. All immunocompromised patients
      ii. Lesions near fovea or optic disc
      iii. Presence of dense vitritis
      iv. Lesions persistent for >1month
      v. Vision significantly reduced from baseline

   c. Triple Therapy

      i. Pyrimethamine: Loading dose of 50 mg BID given 12 hours apart, followed by 25 mg BID dosing
      ii. Sulfadiazine: 2 g BID loading dose, followed by 1 g QiD dosing
      iii. Supplementation with folinic acid: 5 mg twice weekly while taking Pyrimethamine, as the drug can suppress folic acid metabolism

   d. Prednisone 40 mg daily may be started 24–48 hours after antimicrobial therapy with long taper for posterior pole lesions or control of vitritis if severe

e. Clindamycin may be added to form "Quadruple Therapy"

    i. Dosed as 300mg four times daily

    ii. *Important side-effect: Risk of pseudomembranous colitis*

    iii. May also be used as single antimicrobial agent alone or in combination with Trimethoprim–Sulfamethoxazole (1 double strength tablet bid) for patient intolerant to "triple therapy"

f. Azithromycin (250 mg daily) may be used in immunocompotent patients with mild to moderate involvement

g. Atovaquone 750 mg bid for active disease and qd for prophylaxis can be used for patients with sulfa allergies

h. Antimicrobial therapy is continued typically for a minimum of 4 to 6 weeks for immunocompetent patients; indefinite therapy may be indicated for chronically immunocompromised patients

i. All newborns with congenital toxoplasmosis should be treated with antiparasitic medication for the first year of life

j. Long term prophylaxis:

    i. Chronic therapy is indicated in chronically immunosuppressed patients until immune status improves

    ii. Trimethoprim-Sulfamethoxazole (160–800 mg, double strength tablet, every 3 days) may reduce rates of recurrence in immunocompetent patients with posterior pole lesions with history of recurrent disease[3,4]

Syphilis

1. Incidence/Pathophysiology

    a. Caused by spirochete *Treponema pallidum*

    b. Congenital Syphilis occurs in 10 per 100,000 births

    c. Acquired syphilis more common in African American and Homosexual males

    d. Increase in recent incidence secondary to AIDS

    e. Ocular involvement can occur during secondary or tertiary stages

    f. Approximately 5% of patients with untreated secondary syphilis will develop chorioretinitis

2. Clinical Appearance

   a. Placoid Chorioretinitis — single or multiple deep yellow plaques. Which are ill defined and with faded center. May become confluent, often with RPE hyperpigmentation (Figure 3)
   b. Vasculitis, papillitis, neuroretinitis and vitritis also seen in isolation or in association with placoid lesions
   c. Salt-and-pepper pigmentary changes
   d. Known as the Great Masquerader. Should be considered in almost any case of intraocular inflammation[5]

3. Differential Diagnosis:

   a. Acute Posterior Multifocal Placoid Pigmentary Epitheliopathy (APMPPE)
   b. Vogt–Koyanagi–Harada (VKH)
   c. Herpetic retinitis
   d. Toxoplasmosis[6]

4. Diagnostic Testing

   a. Non-treponemal tests: Venereal Disease Research Laboratory (VDRL), rapid plasma reagent (RPR): high sensitivity and low specificity. Usually become nonreactive with time after treatment, may thus be used to track response
   b. Treponemal specific tests: Fluorescent treponemal antibody-absorption (FTA–ABS), microhemagglutination assay *T pallidum* (MHA–TP), *T pallidum* particle agglutination (TPPA). These tests have a high specificity and remain elevated for life. They will not reflect treatment success
   c. Always obtain HIV screening due to high rate of co-infection
   d. Test for neurosyphilis with CSF sent for VDRL/FTA–ABS in all cases of syphilitic uveitis

5. Treatment

   a. Infectious Disease Medical consultation needed
   b. Penicillin G: 10 million units IV daily for 10 days. Gold standard and most effective treatment
   c. Penicillin allergic patients should ideally be desensitized or have concomitant prednisone administration. Alternatively may use doxycycline (100 mg BID) if unable to desensitize
   d. Serum RPR or VDRL can be used to monitor treatment effect

Tuberculosis (TB)

1. Incidence/Pathophysiology

   a. Caused by *Mycobacterium Tuberculosis;* acid-fast obligate aerobe

   b. Represents <1% of uveitis cases in U.S., much higher rates in Africa and Asian countries

   c. Ocular manifestation is typically secondary reactivation of primary pulmonary infection

   d. Higher incidence of ocular manifestation in immunocompromised hosts

2. Clinical Features

   i. Choroidal granuloma or tubercle

   ii. Serpiginous choroidal plaque in posterior pole

   iii. Optic Nerve infiltration with edema

   iv. Periphlebitis and vasculitis

   v. A granulomatous anterior chamber reaction seen in most cases

3. Differential Diagnosis

   a. Serpiginous Choroiditis — more likely to be bilateral and without vitritis

   b. Syphilis

   c. Sarcoidosis

   d. Eale's Disease — peripheral ischemia and vasculitis without vitritis

4. Diagnostic Testing

   a. Tubreculin skin testing (PPD) or Interferron gamma release assays (Qunatiferron Gold)

   b. Chest XRay or CT scan to assess for pulmonary involvement

5. Treatment[7,8]

   a. Treat with multi-drug regimen for at least 6 months

   i. Isoniazid (INH, 300 mg qd)

   ii. Rifampin, 600 mg qd

   iii. Pyrazinamide

   iv. Ethambutol. *Important dose-dependent toxicity is optic neuropathy.*

   v. Supplementation with pyridoxine (B6) 50 mg to prevent neuropathy caused by isoniazid

   vi. Follow liver function test for signs of toxicity to INH and Rifampin

b. Addition of oral steroids should be done shortly after initiation of anti-TB therapy. Typically oral prednisone 1mg/kg with extended taper
c. Referral to Infectious Disease Medical specialist for all suspected cases and Public Health board if active pulmonary disease present

Herpetic Viral Retinochoroiditis

Acute Retinal Necrosis (ARN)

1. Incidence/Etiology

    a. Overall incidence rare: less than 1 per 1 million annually
    b. Most commonly caused by Herpes zoster (HZV), followed by herpes simplex (HSV)
    c. Most commonly occurs in 5th and 6th decades of life

2. Clinical features

    a. Typically unilateral at presentation, 40% bilateral involvement within 6 weeks if untreated (BARN)
    b. Multifocal areas of full-thickness retinal necrosis located in the periphery which spread circumferentially
    c. Prominent vitritis
    d. Stellate Keritatic Precipitates
    e. Papillitis
    f. Occlusive vasculitis with arterial involvement
    g. Typically onset is unilateral, but becomes bilaterally rapidly in majority of patient without treatment
    h. Retinal detachment typically develop due to retinal breaks within necrotic retina

3. Differential Diagnosis

    a. CMV retinitis: Will have perivascular pattern with significant hemorrhages
    b. Disseminated toxoplasma retinochoroiditis
    c. PORN (Progressive outer retinal necrosis)
    d. Syphilis
    e. Behçet disease

4. Diagnostic Testing

    a. Clinical diagnosis is sufficient if classic presentation
    b. Aqueous humor or vitreous PCR may be performed to identify underlying viral pathogen (HZV versus HSV) in atypical cases

c. Assess for history of chickenpox, shingles, herpetic encephalitis, oral herpetic lesions

d. Serum serologic testing for evidence of prior viral exposure

5. Treatment (Table 1)

   a. Intravenous acyclovir is the gold standard for immediate induction of treatment. To be followed by prolonged course of oral acyclovir or valacyclovir. If contraindicated, foscarnet or valganciclovir may be used

   b. For severe vision threatening lesions of the macula and optic nerve, therapy may also include intravitreal foscarnet or ganciclovir

Table 1. Antiviral dosing for herpetic retinochoroiditis.

Induction medication (Given for 10–14 days)

Drug	Dose	Associated Toxicity
Acyclovir	(10 mg/kg/day divided over 3 doses)	Renal dysfunction (Crystalline nephropathy)
Valacyclovir	2 g TID (HZV) PO	Renal dysfunction (Crystalline nephropathy)
Valganciclovir	900mg BID PO	Myelosupression
Foscarnet	90 mg/kg/day divided in 2 doses (ARN) 180 mg/kg/day divided into 2 doses (PORN)	Renal dysfunction

Intravitreal antiviral medications

Drug	Dose
Ganciclovir	200–400 mg/0.1 ml
Foscarnet	1.2–2.4 mg/0.1 ml

Maintenance antiviral medication

Drug	Dose
Acyclovir	800 mg 5 times daily (HZV) 400 mg 5 times daily (HSV)
Valacyclovir	1g TID (HZV) 1g Daily (HSV)
Valganciclovir	900 mg BID
Foscarnet	500 mg BID

    c.   For peripheral lesions, may alternatively induce with oral Valacyclovir for 2 weeks followed by maintenance dosing

    d.   Steroids should be initiated 48 hours after starting antiviral therapy to control optic nerve and intraocular inflammation. If vitiritis dense, consider starting with IV solumedrol 250 mg BID followed by oral prednisone starting at 1 mg/kg/day. May start directly with oral prednisone in less severe cases. Prolonged taper is necessary to prevent rebound vitritis

    e.   Duration of long-term anti-viral treatment is uncertain, but should extend at least 3 months. Chronic therapy is indicated in immunosuppressive patients

    f.   Aspirin (325 mg daily) may be used to prevent intraretinal vascular occlusion[9,10]

Progressive Outer Retinal Necrosis (PORN)

1. Pathophysiology/Incidence

    a.   A variant of ARN seen in immunocompromised patients
    b.   Typically seen in AIDS patients with CD 4<50
    c.   Overwhelming majority of cases are from HZV

2. Clinical features

    a.   Lesions appear similar to ARN, but may be seen in posterior pole at onset and tends to spread in outward fashion
    b.   Vitritis and anterior chamber reaction are usually mild to absent
    c.   Majority will have bilateral involvement

3. Diagnostic testing

    a.   Clinical diagnosis typically
    b.   Aqueous PCR and IgM may be obtained to confirm presence of HZV
    c.   MRI Brain and lumbar puncture should be obtained due to high rate of concomitant encephalitis in immunocompromised patients

4. Differential Diagnosis: similar to ARN
5. Treatment

    a.   PORN is normally resistant to intravenous acyclovir alone
    b.   Intravitreal foscarnet or ganciclovir is necessary in most cases
    c.   Immune reconstitution must be achieved in AIDS patients in order to discontinue long-term antiviral treatment

d. Unlike with ARN, steroids and anti-inflammatories should be avoided since patients are already immunocompromised

e. Even with adequate treatment, visual prognosis remains very poor

Cytomegalovirus (CMV)

1. Pathophysiology/Incidence

   a. Occur primarily in immunosuppressed individuals

      i. AIDS with CD4+ < 50; may lead to initial diagnosis of AIDS in 15% of patients.[11] Responsible for over 40% of HIV-related vision loss[12]

      ii. Solid-organ transplant patients

   b. Retinal Detachment may occur in 30% of patients, often with multiple, hidden retinal breaks within the area of old retinitis[13]

2. Clinical Features (Figure 4)

   a. Slowly progressive necrotizing hemorrhagic retinitis

   b. Multiple, confluent, yellow-white areas with interspersed overlying prominent retinal hemorrhages

   c. Perivascular inflammation (sometimes frosted-branch angiitis)

   d. Sharp demarcation between involved and healthy retina

   e. Vitritis typically minimal

   f. Sight threatening if Zone I disease (within 2 disc-diameters of fovea or optic nerve)

3. Differential diagnoses

   a. Other herpetic retinochoroiditis (ARN/PORN)

   b. Idiopathic frosted branch angiitis

   c. Intraocular lymphoma

4. Diagnostic testing

   a. Given the typical appearance, no confirmatory testing is generally necessary except serum serologic testing to confirm prior viral exposure (high rate of sero-positivity in the general adult population)

   b. PCR from aqueous or vitreous may be helpful in atypical presentation

   c. Establish Systemic CMV viral load

   d. Obtain Infectious Disease consult

   e. If HIV status unknown; HIV screen, HIV viral load, CD4+

5. Treatment

   a. Systemic antiviral therapy (Table 2)

       i. Valganciclovir is treatment of choice since orally administered but good ocular penetration

           1. Important side effects: neutropenia and thrombocytopenia. May be contraindicated in select patients and alternate therapy may be considered

       ii. Maintenance medication should be continued until immune reconstitution present for at least 6 months

   b. Intravitreal Treatment

       i. Given in all patients with Zone I disease resistant to systemic antiviral therapy
       ii. Treatment should be given 2 times weekly for at least 2 weeks
       iii. Ganciclovir intravitreal implant (4.5 mg) is no longer available

   c. If treatment with ganciclovir or valganciclovir appears to be ineffective, alternative antiviral therapy should be considered. Genetic testing is available to test for drug resistance of the virus

Table 2.   Systemic and intravitreal medical therapy for Cytomegalovirus retinitis.

Systemic dosing in CMV retinitis.

Drug	Induction*	Maintenance
Valganciclovir*	900 mg BID PO for 3 weeks	900 mg PO Daily
Ganciclovir	5 mg/kg BID IV	5 mg/kg daily
Cidofovir	5 mg/kg weekly	5 mg/kg q^2 weeks
Foscarnet	90 mg/kg/day BID	500 mg BID

* Administered for 2 weeks.

Intravitreal medication in CMV retinitis.

Drug	Dose
Ganciclovir	2.5 mg/0.05 ml
Foscarnet	1.2 mg/0.05 ml

d. Recurrent disease should be treated with similar induction course as with initial episode

e. Ensure HAART has been initiated (immune recovery is paramount to help resolve CMV retinitis)[14]

Management of Retinal Detachment associated with Viral Retintis ARN/PORN/ CMV retinitis

- *Detachments are repaired with vitrectomy, endolaser and placement of silicone oil to tamponade necrotic and diaphanous retina*
- *No role for primary scleral buckling*
- *Laser does not halt advancement of necrosis, but does have benefit in preventing retinal detachment and may be employed to surround visible breaks[13,15]*

Refer to Chapter 24 on Retinal Detachment for more details

Presumed Ocular Histoplasmosis Syndrome (POHS)

1. Incidence/Pathophysiology

   a. Most common in Ohio and Mississippi river valleys

   b. Not a clear causal relationship to the fungus *Histoplasma capsulatum*, but epidemiologically correlated

   c. Likely an immune-mediate response to previous fungus exposure

   d. Prevalence varies geographically: 1–2% of general population in endemic areas have asymptomatic scars

   e. Development of ocular lesions is less than less than 1% per year

2. Clinical Features

   a. Discrete, well-demarcated chorioretinal scars ("punched-out" lesions)

   b. Peripapillary atrophy

   c. Choroidal neovascularization (CNVM) with subretinal hemorrhage, exudates, eventual disciform scarring.

   d. Peripheral circumferential linear pigment streaks (5%)

   e. Absence of vitreous cells[16]

3. Differential Diagnosis

   a. Punctate Inner Choroidopathy

   b. Multifocal Choroiditis; will typically have more robust vitreous and AC reaction

   c. Age-Related Macula Degeneration

   d. TB[17]

4. Diagnostic Testing

   a. POHS is universally a clinical diagnosis based on above features
   b. Histoplasma skin testing is usually not performed due to low specificity
   c. Macular OCT to screen to macular fluid to rule out active CNVM
   d. Fluorescein angiography if suspicion for CNVM on exam or OCT

5. Treatment

   a. Only macular lesions with CNVM require treatment as peripheral histo spots are not visually significant
   b. Anti-VEGF therapy has been shown effective for vision threatening CNVM
   c. *Macular Photocoagulation Study* demonstrated that thermal laser may be utilized for extrafoveal and some juxtafoveal CNVM
   d. *Photodynamic therapy may also be used alone or in combination with anti-VEGF therapy for subfoveal CNVM*
   e. Submacular surgery for subfoveal lesions with poor vision (<20/100) if disease is recalcitrant to all other treatments
   f. Patients should be instructed on Amsler grid use for monitoring of CNVM

Toxocara

1. Incidence/Pathophysiology

   a. Caused by helminth *Toxocara Canis*
   b. Typically transmitted through fecal–oral contamination and exposure to dogs and cats
   c. Average age of onset is 7–8 years

2. Clinical features
3. Principal clinical forms which are age-dependent at presentation

   a. Posterior pole granuloma: Ages 6–14. Solitary yellow–white granuloma in posterior fundus, minimal inflammation. May cause tractional detachment or epiretinal membrane
   b. Peripheral granulomas: Age 15 and above. may be solitary or multifocal, with prominent vitreous band extending to optic disc
   c. Chronic endophthalmitis: Ages 2–9. Leukocoria, dense vitreous opacities, granulomatous AC reaction
   d. Al forms are almost universally unilateral[18]

3. Differential Diagnosis

   a. Retinoblastoma: leukokorea but will not have significant inflammatory component and will demonstrate growth
   b. Retinopathy of prematurity
   c. Coats
   d. Familial Exudative Vitreoretinopathy (FEVR)
   e. Persistent Fetal Vasculature (PFV)
   f. Bacterial or Fungal endophthalmitis
   g. Tuberculosis granuloma

4. Diagnostic Testing

   a. Serum antibodies have low sensitivity, aqueous and vitreous ELISA for IgM is more sensitive if clinical picture is uncertain
   b. Peripheral eosinophilia is suggestive
   c. B scan ultrasonography is essential to assess for tractional components in presence of significant media opacity

5. Treatment

   a. Antihelminth therapy may not be necessary as ocular pathology is primarily an inflammatory reaction. The most common therapy is Albendazole 10 mg/kg/day
   b. Systemic and periocular steroids are mainstay of treatment
   c. Topical cycloplegics and steroids may be employed for anterior chamber inflammation
   d. Tractional retinal detachments, epiretinal membranes and fibrous bands are repaired typically with Pars Plana Vitrecotmy

References

1. Holland GN. Ocular toxoplasmosis: A global reassessment: Part I: Epidemiology and course of disease. *Am J Ophthalmol* 2003;136:973–988.

2. Holland GN. Ocular toxoplasmosis: A global reassessment: part II: disease manifestations and management. *Am J Ophthalmol* 2004;137:1–17.

3. Kim SJ, Scott IU, Brown GC, *et al.* Interventions for toxoplasma retinochoroiditis: A report by the american academy of ophthalmology. *Ophthalmol* 2013;120:371–378.

4. Soheilian M, Sadoughi M-M, Ghajarnia M, *et al.* Prospective randomized trial of trimethoprim/sulfamethoxazole versus pyrimethamine and sulfadiazine in the treatment of ocular toxoplasmosis. *Ophthalmol* 2005;112:1876–1882.

5. Browning DJ. Posterior segment manifestations of active ocular syphilis, their response to a neurosyphilis regimen of penicillin therapy, and the influence of human immunodeficiency virus status on response. *Ophthalmol* 2000;107:2015–2023.

6. Kiss Sr, Damico FM, Young LH. Ocular manifestations and treatment of syphilis. *Seminars Ophthalmol* 2005;20:161–167.

7. Bansal R, Gupta A, Gupta V, *et al.* Role of anti-tubercular therapy in uveitis with latent/manifest tuberculosis. *Am J Ophthalmol* 2008;146:772–779.

8. Cutrufello NJ, Karakousis PC, Fishler J, *et al.* Intraocular tuberculosis. *Ocul Immunol Inflamm* 2010;18:281–291.

9. Aizman A, Johnson MW, Elner SG. Treatment of acute retinal necrosis syndrome with oral antiviral medications. *Ophthalmol* 2007;114:307–312.

10. Tibbetts MD, Shah CP, Young LH, *et al.* Treatment of acute retinal necrosis. *Ophthalmol* 2010;117:818–824.

11. Sison RF HG, MacArthur LJ, *et al.* Cytomegalovirus retinopathy as the initial manifestation of the acquired immunodeficiency syndrome. *Am J Ophthalmol* 1991;112:243–249.

12. Thorne JE, Holbrook JT, Jabs DA, *et al.* Effect of cytomegalovirus retinitis on the risk of visual acuity loss among patients with AIDS. *Ophthalmol* 2007;114:591–598.

13. Althaus C, Loeffler KU, Schimkat M, *et al.* Prophylactic argon laser coagulation for rhegmatogenous retinal detachment in AIDS patients with cytomegalovirus retinitis. *Graefes Arch Clin Exp Ophthalmol* 1998;236:359–364.

14. Barrett L, Walmsley S. CMV retinopathy in the antiretroviral therapy era: Prevention, diagnosis and management. *Curr Infect Dis Rep* 2012;14:435–444.

15. Stevens G. Failure of argon laser to halt cytomegalovirus retinitis. *Retina* 1986;6:119–122.

16. Ganley JP SR, Knox DL, Comstock GW. Presumed ocular histoplasmosis. 3. epidemiologic characteristics of people with peripheral atrophic scars. *Arch Ophthalmol* 1973;89:116–119.

17. Smith RE GJ. The natural history of non-disciform ocular histoplasmosis. *Can J Ophthalmol* 1977;12:114–120.

18. Stewart JM, Cunningham, E.T. Prevalence, clinical features and causes of visual loss among patients with ocular toxocariasis. *Retina* 2005;25:1005–1013.

19. Nusunblatt RB WS. Uveitis: Fundamentals and Clinical Practice. Fourth Edition. St. Louis: Mosby, 2010.

Chapter 21: Endophthalmitis

Senad Osmanovic and Susanna S. Park

Post-Surgical

1. Incidence varies depending on procedure and associated risk factors:

    a) Procedure:

        a. Cataract Extraction

            i. Phacoemulsification versus Extracapsular 0.04–0.07%

        b. Filtering Bleb: 0.06%
        c. Glaucoma Drainage Implant: ~2%

            i. associated with exposure of implant

        d. Corneal Transplant: 0.11%
        e. Pars-Plana Vitrectomy: ~ 0.05%
        f. Intravitreal Injection ~0.06%

    b) Intra-cameral antibiotics during cataract surgery may reduce infection rates
    c) Risk Factors: blepharitis, nasolacrimal duct obstruction, prolonged surgery or intraoperative complications (capsular tear, vitreous loss), postoperative wound leak or suture abscess, diabetic or immunocompromised patient (HIV, malignancy)

2. Clinical Features and Findings

    a) Acute endophthalmitis

        a. Acute onset of redness, pain and reduced vision
        b. Typically occurs 1–6 days after procedure

        c.   Progressive vitritis is hallmark

        d.   Hypopyon/ Fibrin in anterior chamber

        e.   Corneal edema may be seen

        f.   Look for presence of contributing lesions, such as wound leak, suture abscess, vitreous prolapse to wound, eroding scleral sutures, exposed drainage tubing, etc.

  b) Chronic endophthalmitis

        a.   Vision loss and inflammation are more indolent and subtle

           i.   Occurs > 6 weeks following surgery

        b.   Presence of posterior capsular plaque

        c.   Chronic recurrent low grade vitritis

        d.   Inflammation may occur as late as 2 years following cataract surgery

        e.   Inflammation may be precipitated by YAG posterior capsulotomy

3. Etiology: may varying depending on procedure

  a) Post cataract surgery causes:

          i. *Coagulase Negative Staphylococcus* (CNS) 65%

        ii. *Staph aureus* 10%

       iii. *Streptococcus* species 10%

       iv. Culture-negative cases can account for 15–30% of cases

  b) Keratoplasty and Keratoprosthesis: gram negative organisms, fungal and protazoal etiologies are rare but increasingly common in this setting

  c) Following Intravitreal injection:

          i. Coagulase-negative *Staph* 38%

        ii. *Strep.* Species are second most common (30%)

  d) Filtering Blebs: >50% *Streptococcus* species

  e) Chronic post operative endophthalmitis (> 6 weeks)

          i. *Propionibacterium acnes* most common following cataract surgery

        ii. Other causes less common

4. Diagnostic Testing

  a) B-scan Ultrasonography (Figure 1)

          i. No diagnostic findings for acute endophthalmitis but important test to rule out retinal detachment or abscess, which may alter management

    ii. Presence of vitreous echogenicity does not diagnose endophalmitis but increased echogenicity compare with fellow eye may suggest vitreous inflammation

    iii. Presence of tractional membranes are suggestive of acute endophthalmitis especially if new

b) Vitreous Biopsy

    i. Done either as tap or via vitrectomy

    ii. In acutely inflamed eyes it may be difficult to obtain vitreous tap due to increased vitreous viscosity

        i. A larger gauge needle (≥ 25 g) and syringe (3 cc syringe) may allow for more vacuum pressure

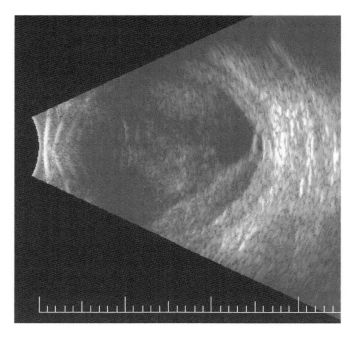

Figure 1. B-scan ultrasonography of an eye with severe intraocular inflammation from endopthalmitis following intravitreal injection showing diffuse choroidal thickening and a focal preretinal hyperreflective mass. Vitrectomy was performed which revealed this preretinal lesion to be a pre-retinal abscess.

   iii. If unable to obtain vitreous sample, perform anterior chamber paracentesis to obtain aqueous sample

      i. minimum 0.2 cc

   iv. If vitrectomy is used, sample should be obtained prior to irrigation being turned on to obtain undiluted specimen

   v. Corneal cultures may be also obtained if corneal infiltrate or abscess is noted and thought to be source

   vi. Positive cultures may only be seen in 60 to 75% of cases

5. Differential Diagnosis

  a) Post-operative inflammation

    i) Responds to corticosteroid but may worsen with corticosteroid taper

  b) Toxic anterior segment syndrome

    i) Typically seen < 24hrs following anterior segment surgery
    ii) Caused by toxicity to irrigation solution contaminants during surgery
    iii) Treated with topical corticosteroid

  c) Large cell lymphoma

    i) May simulate chronic endophthalmitis/vitritis

6. Treatment

Key Study: Endophthalmitis Vitrectomy Study (EVS)
EVS evaluated acute postoperative (<6 weeks following surgery) endophthalmitis following cataract extraction or secondary IOL implantation. Results may serve as general guideline for postoperative endophthalmitis, but may not apply directly to exogenous endophthalmitis associated with other surgeries or injections, post-traumatic and endogenous endophthalmitis

  Summary of findings:

• Patients with HM visions or better visual acuity at presentation did equally well with intravitreal injection of antibiotics regardless of whether pars planar vitrectomy was performed at presentation acutely. Eyes with LP vision at presentation did better if vitrectomy was performed acutely before intrvitreal injection of antibiotics

• Addition of systemic antibiotics (ceftazidime and amikacin) did not result in improved visual outcomes. However, there is controversy as to whether this combination of systemic antiobiotics was ideal choice for treating endophthalmitis

a) Antibiotics

   i. Intravitreal administration is mainstay of therapy

      1. Broad spectrum coverage with minimal toxicity

      2. Table 1 summarizes the intravitreal doses of antibiotics that can be used

         a. Vancomycin and ceftazidime is the most commonly used combination in an acute setting

   ii. Systemic antibiotics

      1. EVS found no difference in outcomes with systemic antibiotics (ceftazidime and amikacin). However, these agents may not have been the ideal choice of antibiotics for systemic administration

      2. Oral 4th generation floroquinalones may be used as adjunct therapy given good intraocular penetration, broad coverage, and low risk profile

         a. Example: moxifloxacin 400 mg daily

b) Pars Plana Vitrectomy

   i. Indications based on EVS: LP presenting vision, presence of retinal detachment

   ii. For chronic *P. acnes* infection, vitrectomy may be indicated in order to at least partially remove the lens capsule

Table 1. Common intravitreal medications for treatment of endophthalmitis.

Medication	Dose
Ceftazidime	2.25 mg/0.1 ml
Cefazolin	2.25 mg/0.1 ml
Vancomycin	1 mg/0.1 ml
Amikacin	400 mg/0.1 ml
Amphoteracin	10 mg/0.1 ml
Voriconazole	100 mg/0.1 ml
Dexamethasone	0.4 mg/0.1 ml

Intravitreal injection antibacterial agents are typically effective in >MIC concentrations for 24 to 48 hours.[18]

   iii. May be indicated for nonclearing vitreous opacity or debris or persistent inflammation following intravitreal antiobiotic treatment

c) Intravitreal Corticosteroid

   a. Dexamethasone 0.4 mg/0.1 cc:

      i. Typically used since short acting (few hours)

      ii. May inhibit the inflammatory effects of bacterial endotoxins and minimize the inflammatory damage to the retina associated with the bactericidal effects of antibiotic treatment

      iii. No adverse effect has been reported clinically but use is somewhat controversial as conflicting results have been reported on improvement of visual outcomes

      iv. Use was not evaluated in EVS; all patients received *systemic prednisone*

      v. In animal model of pneumococcal endophthamitis, intravitreal dexamethasone dramatically preserved the retinal anatomy and decreased elimination of intravitreal vancomycin

      vi. Intravitreal dexamethasone (400 µg) during initial antibiotic administration may be considered in cases of robust inflammation at presentation especially when infection is associated with more virulent organisms

d) Topical treatment

   a. Cycloplegia

      i. Initiate as soon as possible for comfort and to minimize synechiae

   b. Corticosteroid

      i. Initiate at least qid following antibiotic treatment to control inflammation

   c. Broad-spectrum antiobiotics

      i. Fortified antiobiotics or fluoroquinolone with good ocular penetration recommended

      ii. Aggressive therapy every 1 to 2 hours during the acute management with taper pending response

e) Follow-up care

  i. Should be seen daily following initial presentation and treatment
  ii. Monitor level of pain

    a. Best early gauge of treatment response as sterilized eyes should have significant improvement in pain as soon as 24 hours after intravitreal antibiotic injection

  iii. Repeat intravitreal antibiotic injection and/or vitrectomy can be considered after 36–48 hours if pain persists or inflammation continues to worsens
  iv. In EVS, 10% of patients underwent additional procedure within 1st week (mainly for increasing inflammation); 27% had late procedures — removal of lens/capsule, retinal detachment repair or glaucoma surgery

7. Prognosis

  a) Visual outcomes are better in culture negative cases, coagulase-negative *Staph* and with *P. acnes* as the etiologic agent. Outcomes worse with *Strep* Species
  b) The rates of achieving final visual acuity of 20/100 or better are dependent on organism: Gram-positive, coagulase-negative micrococci, 84%; Gram-negative organisms, 14%; *Staphylococcus aureus*, 50%; *Streptococci*, 30%; and *Enterococci*, 14% (EVS study)
  c) In the Endophthalmitis Vitrectomy Study 33% of eyes with initial vision of light perception achieved 20/40 when treated with immediate vitrectomy, 56% achieved 20/100 (versus 30%). In eyes with HM or better vision, over 60% of such eyes achieved 20/40 or better visual acuity regardless of whether vitrectomy was performed

Post-Traumatic Endophthalmitis

1. Incidence

  a) Endophthalmitis following penetrating trauma: 3.3% to 17%

b) Intraocular foreign body (IOFB) increases endophthalmitis incidence

    i. 11–30% especially if trauma involving organic material

    ii. Risk increases if there is violation of lens capsule as well

c) Risk increased with delayed presentation following injury (>24 hours)

2. Clinical Features

    a) Presentation similar to post-operative endophthalmitis

    b) Important to differentiate from inflammation due to trauma

3. Etiology

    a) Polymicrobial infection more common — over 40% may have multiple pathogens

    b) Gram Positive Species still predominate:

        i. Higher rates of *S. aureus* and *Strep* species than postoperative cases

    c) High incidence of *Bacillus* species, particularly *B. cereus.*

        i. 40% of trauma involving soil/organic matter

        ii. Bacillus species are very aggressive, with extensive necrosis of tissues evident by 24–48 hours — majority of eyes result in complete vision loss

4. Diagnostic Testing:

    a) CT to rule out IOFB (Intraocular foreign body)

        i. MRI avoided in instances of suspected metal element

    b) Important to exclude occult IOFB that is not seen on initial imaging if persistent ocular inflammation is noted after open globe repair

        i. Consider Echography (B Scan, UBM)

    c) Vitreous and aqueous cultures should be obtained in all suspected cases during the time of globe repair

5. Therapy

    a) Pars planar vitrectomy

        i. Threshold to undergo immediate vitrectomy is low in this setting as there is a higher incidence of more severe organisms resulting in poorer visual prognosis

      ii. Concomitant lensectomy should be performed if lens capsule is violated

      iii. Removal of any IOFB present is essential and must be done in emergent manner if present

  b) Intravitreal antibiotics

      i. Broad spectrum coverage as soon as globe repair and/or vitrectomy is completed

      ii. Selection of antibiotics similar to post-operative endophthalmitis

      iii. Antibiotics should not be narrowed due to increased presence of polymicrobial infections

  c) Intravitreal corticosteroid (Dexamethasone)

      i. Although there is limited data on this, given the risk of more virulent organisms that might be associated, intravitreal dexamethasone should be considered at the time of intravitreal antibiotic administration

6. Follow-up care

  a) Similar to post-operative endophthalmitis, almost daily follow up during early course is needed till patient shows clinical improvement

7. Prognosis

  a) Overall prognosis is worse than in post-operative setting, owing to more severe spectrum of bacterial pathogens

  b) Only 27% achieved acuity of 20/400; this likely reflects effect of initial trauma

Endogenous Endophthalmitis

1. Incidence

  a) Endogenous Bacterial Endophthalmitis (EBE) represents less than 8% of all endophthalmitis cases

      i. Largest predisposing risk factor is active infection elsewhere in body (i.e. pneumonia, endocarditis, bacteremia, Liver abscess)

      ii. Patients at risk for transient bacteremia;

          1. Intravenous drug users

      2. Recent procedure: dental surgery, endoscopy/colonoscopy, invasive angiography

b) Fungal Endophthalmitis

    i. Endogenous infection is the most common setting for fungal endophthalmitis

    ii. Risk Factors for fungemia: IV hyperalimentation, long-term antibiotic usage, GI surgery, cancer surgery, diabetes

    iii. 30% incidence of ocular involvement following fungemia if no anti-fungal therapy is given

    iv. 2–3% risk of chorioretinitis/endophthalmitis following fungemia in setting of anti-fungal therapy

    v. Risk Factors for Ocular Fungal involvement

        1. Visual Symptoms

        2. Persistent fungemia despite anti-fungal treatment

        3. Immunosuppression (HIV, malignancy)

2. Etiology

a) Bacteria

    i. Streptococcus species (Group B primarily) ~30%

    ii. *Staph* aureus 10–20%

    iii. Gram Negative (*Pseudomonas, Neisseria, E. Coli*) 30–50%

    iv. *Klebsiella Pneumoniae* is associated with liver abscess. More common is East Asia or Asian immigrants

b) Fungal

    i. *Candida* species and *Aspergillus* species most common

    ii. *Candida Albicans accounts for* ~50%

    iii. *Candida Kruzei* emerging due to resistance to fluconazole

    iv. *Cryptococcus Neoformans* common in HIV population

3. Clinical Features and Findings

a) Any significant past medical or travel history should be documented

b) As a rule, bilateral involvement should raise suspicion for endogenous endophthalmitis

c) Bacterial infection

    i. Dense Vitritis

    ii. Subretinal abscesses (*Pseudomonas, Klebsiella*)

    iii. Layered abscess may be seen in *Nocardia* infections ("*Retinal pseudohypopyon*"); seen in immunocompromised patients with pneumonia

    iv. May have associated Roths spots—emboli from septic nidus

d) Fungal (Figure 2)

    i. Yellow white, deep chorioretinal lesions

    ii. Vitreous fluff balls ("string of pearls")

    iii. *Candida* species tend to demonstrate grater vitreous involvement. *Aspergillus* species tend to have isolate chorioretinal lesions. Overall more indolent course compared to bacterial infections

4. Diagnostic Studies

a) In cases of unknown source of infection, a thorough systemic work up should be performed

    i. Blood and Urine Cultures

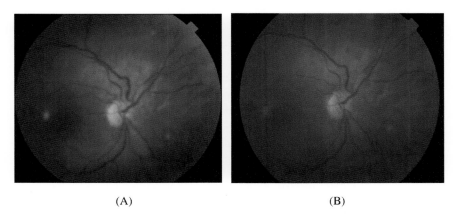

(A)   (B)

Figure 2. (A) Fundus photograph of the right eye with early multifocal retinochoroiditis and vitritis from *candida fungemia*. (B) One month after intravitreal amphotericin and oral fluconazole therapy, the intraocular infection is resolved leaving small focal scars.

ii. Echocardiography

    1. trans-esophageal imaging may be needed to visualize cardiac valve lesions

iii. Chest X-ray or CT

iv. Abdominal Ultrasound or MRI/CT imaging to evaluate for liver abscess

    1. high rate of liver abscess in *Klebsiella* endophthalmitis

v. Infectious disease consultation is essential and should be sought early in course

vi. Testing for HIV status if not known

b) B scan ultrasonography of the eye should be employed if media opacity prevents reliable assessment of retina

    i. Evaluate for presence of abscess, tractional membranes or retinal detachment

c) Vitreous and aqueous biopsy for culture

    i. Important especially if no unknown source of infection

    ii. May be deferred if organism has been identified by blood culture

5. Treatment

a) Bacterial Infection:

    i. Systemic antibiotics (intravenous) are imperative to treat underlying nidus of infection. Broad spectrum coverage should be initiated first, such as a combination of vancomycin and 3rd or 4th generation cephalosporin or aminoglycoside

    ii. Intravitreal antibiotics should be utilized unless clinical picture is subtle or uncertain

        1. Trend towards globe preservation with local combined with systemic antimicrobial therapy

        2. Choice of antibacterial agent similar to post-operative endophthalmitis–vancomycin and ceftazidime most popular

    iii. Early vitrectomy in setting of subretinal abscess which may not respond to systemic or intravitreal therapy

b) Fungal Infection

   i. Systemic antifungals are mainstay

      1. Fluconazole (*Candida*) or Voriconazole (*Candida/ Aspergillus*) have excellent ocular penetration
      2. Amphoteracin B: Should be reserved in recalcitrant cases due to the increased severity of side-effects such as fever, hypotension, hepatotoxicity

   ii. Intravitreal Antifungal

      1. Voriconazole or Amphotericin
      2. Indicated for progressive vitritis or vision threatening disease

6. Prognosis

   a) Variable depending on etiology of infection

      i. Bacterial cases: > 50% of eyes may have vision worse than 20/200. Overall outcome and rates of enucleation are less favorable than for post-operative scenario
      ii. Fungal cases: prognosis highly dependent on timing of treatment initiation and macular involvement

Surgical Considerations and Pearls

Disclaimer: The Endophthalmitis Vitrectomy Study (EVS) specifically looked at acute post-operative endophthalmitis. As such, thresholds for Vitrectomy in setting of post-traumatic and enodgenous endophthalmitis maybe lower due to a different and more severe microbial spectrum.

1. General Anesthesia is preferred due to the difficulty in obtaining effective local anesthesia in an acutely inflamed eye
2. During vitrectomy setup, it may be difficult to confirm the intravitreal position of the infusion cannula initially as there is often significant media opacity in the anterior chamber from hypopyon or corneal edema. Insertion of infusion cannula and vitrector through an anterior chamber paracentesis may be necessary prior to obtaining a view for pars plana instrumentation

3. In phakic eyes, lensectomy may be considered if the lens is opacified or there is significant inflammatory debris around the lens capsule precluding adequate fundus visualization. In pseudophakic eyes, the lens implant may be kept in place if view is cleared with capsulotomy

4. In eyes with a totally opacified cornea, a temporary keratoprosthesis may be necessary

5. An undiluted sample of vitreous and/or aqueous fluid should be obtained for culture before infusion is started in the eye

6. Retina is often necrotic and removal of inflammatory membranes and/or adherent vitreous may result in retinal breaks and detachments easily

7. Using gas or oil tamponade makes use of intravitreal antibiotic administration more difficult as it may result in variable distribution and higher than desired concentration of medication

References

1. Eifrig CW FH, Scott IU, *et al*. Acute-onset postoperative endophthalmitis: Review of incidence and visual outcomes. *Ophthalmol Surg Lasers* 2002;33:373–378.
2. Kattan HM FH, Pflugfelder SC, *et al*. Nosocomia endophthalmitis survey: Current incidence of infection following intraocular surgery. *Ophthalmol* 1991;98:227238.
3. Christakis PG, Tsai JC, Kalenak JW, *et al*. The Ahmed Versus Baerveldt Study: Three-Year Treatment Outcomes. *Ophthalmol* 2013;120:2232–2240.
4. Fileta JB, Flynn HW. Meta-analysis of infectious endophthalmitis after intravitreal injection of anti-vascular endothelial growth factor agents. *Ophthalmic Surg Laser and Imaging Retina* 2014;45:143–149.
5. Garcia-Saenz MC, Arias-Puente A, Rodriguez-Caravaca G, *et al*. Effectiveness of intracameral cefuroxime in preventing endophthalmitis after cataract surgery: Ten-year comparative study. *J Cataract Refractive Surg* 2010;36:203–207.
6. Benz MS, Scott IU, Flynn Jr HW, *et al*. Endophthalmitis isolates and antibiotic sensitivities: A 6-year review of culture-proven cases. *Am J Ophthalmol* 2004;137: 38–42.
7. Kangas TA FH. Delayed-onset endophthalmitis assciated with conjunctival filtering blebs. *Ophthalmol* 1997;104:746–752.
8. Results of the endophthalmitis vitrectomy study: A randomized trial of immediate vitrectomy and of intravenous antibiotics for the treatment of postoperative bacterial endophthalmitis. *Arch Ophthalmol* 1995;113:1479–1496.
9. Clark WL, Kaiser PK, Flynn Jr HW, *et al*. Treatment strategies and visual acuity outcomes in chronic postoperative propionibacterium acnes endophthalmitis. *Ophthalmol* 1999;106:1665–1670.
10. Dev S HD, Mieler WF, *et al*. The role of intravitreal dexamethasone as an adjunct in the management of postoperative bacterial endophthalmitis. *J Eur Vitreoretinal Soc* 2004:13–20.
11. Shah GK SJ, Sharma S, *et al*. Visual outcomes following the use of intravitreal steroids in the treatment of postoperative endophthalmitis. *Ophthalmol* 2000;107:486–489.
12. Park SS, Vallar RV, Hong C, *et al*. Intravitreal dexamethasone effect on intravitreal vancomycin elimination in endophthalmitis. *Arch Ophthalmol* 1999;117:1058–1062.
13. Meredith TA. Post-traumatic endophthalmitis. *Arch Ophthalmol* 1999;117:520–521.
14. Soheilian M, Rafati N, Mohebbi M, *et al*. Prophylaxis of acute posttraumatic bacterial endophthalmitis: A multicenter, randomized clinical trial of intraocular antibiotic injection, Report 2. *Arch Ophthalmol* 2007;125:460–465.
15. Boldt HC PJ, Blodi CF, Weingeist TA. Rural endophthalmitis. *Ophthalmol* 1989;96:1722–1726.
16. Scherer WJ, Lee K. Implications of early systemic therapy on the incidence of endogenous fungal endophthalmitis. *Ophthalmol* 1997;104:1593–1598.
17. Jackson TL, Paraskevopoulos T, Georgalas I. Systematic review of 342 cases of endogenous bacterial endophthalmitis. *Surv Ophthalmol* 2014;59:627–635.

18. Riddell J, Comer GM, Kauffman CA. Treatment of endogenous fungal endophthalmitis: Focus on new antifungal agents. *Clin Infect Dis* 2011;52:648–653.
19. Park SS, Samily N, Ruoff K, D'Amico DJ, Sullivan Baker A. Effect of intravitreal dexamethasone in treatment of pneumococcal endophthalmitis in rabbits. *Arch Ophthalmol* 1995;113:1324–1329.
20. Yang CS, Tsai HY, Sung Cs, *et al*. Endogenous klebsiella endophthalmitis associated with pyogenic liver abscess. *Ophthalmol* 2007;114:876–880.

SECTION 6: TRAUMA

Chapter 22: Surgical Management of Posterior Segment Trauma

Eric K. Chin, David R.P. Almeida and Susanna S. Park

Indications for Urgent Vitreo-retinal Surgical Intervention:

1. Intraocular Foreign Body (IOFB)

a. Background

   i. Risk factors = male, young/middle-aged

   ii. Present in up to 40% of traumatic ocular injury cases

   iii. CT is considered the gold standard imaging technique for acute orbital foreign body

      1. Plastic, wood and fish bones are radiolucent on CT

      2. Wood can be mistaken for air on CT

b. Variables fostering poor prognosis

   i. Poor initial VA

   ii. Large IOFB size

   iii. Posterior segment location

   iv. Pre-operative retinal detachment

c. Which foreign bodies are greatest risk and why should they be removed

   i. Poorly tolerated

      1. Organic (e.g. wood, vegetable matter)

      2. Chemical (e.g. diesel fuel)

      3. Retinotoxic metallic foreign bodies (especially copper)

    4. Magnetic (e.g. iron, steel and tin)

    5. Non-magnetic (e.g. copper and vegetable matter)

  ii. Fairly well tolerated

    1. Alloys that are <85% copper (e.g. bronze, brass)

    2. Magnetic (e.g. nickel)

    3. Non-magnetic (e.g. aluminum, mercury, zinc)

  iii. Inert foreign bodies

    1. Glass, lead, plastics

d. Surgical equipment for IOFB removal

  i. 20-gauge versus 23-gauge vitrectomy often required

    1. Foreign body forceps (e.g. non-magnetic foreign bodies)

    2. Intraocular magnet (e.g. magnetic IOFB)

    3. Scissors, pick or Tano scraper for membrane removal (e.g. when IOFB is encapsulated)

    4. Fragmatome (e.g. dense dropped lens material)

    5. MVR blade to enlarge opening for prolapse of IOFB (size-dependent)

  ii. Alternative sources of illumination, such as a chandelier light or illuminated pick, to allow for bimanual surgery

  iii. Perfluorocarbon (PFO) liquid may be used to avoid iatrogenic subretinal hemorrhage and decrease the possible traumatic impact of a foreign body falling on the macula during removal

  iv. Scleral buckling may reduce the risk of late onset retinal detachment (6.6% retinal detachment with a scleral buckle, versus 30.8% without a scleral buckle, $P = 0.24$)

2. Traumatic Endophthalmitis

a. Background

  i. Incidence of culture-positive endophthalmitis after open globe repair seen in 1.9%

  ii. Associated with poor visual outcome and hypotony

  iii. Comprises of 25–31% of all infectious endophthalmitis

b. Clinical presentation

    i. Decreased or worsening vision and/or pain

    ii. Hypopyon, vitritis, retinal periphlebitis, corneal ring infiltrate, panophthalmitis

    iii. Rapid onset (often <24 hours) especially with more virulent organisms

c. Factors associated with endophthalmitis

    i. Dirty wound

        1. Bilateral ocular trauma (2.9%) seen with blast injuries

    ii. Rural setting, related to higher incidence of soil contamination.

    iii. Delayed presentation or wound closure (>24 hours)

        1. Four-fold increase in infection rate when delay of >24 hours

    iv. Retained IOFB

        1. Incidence varies from 6.9 to 16.5%

    v. Disruption of crystalline lens gives microorganism direct access to the vitreous cavity as well as impedes their clearance by blocking the normal flow of aqueous and may also serve as a source of nutrition for growth of microorganism

    vi. Primary intraocular lens placement

d. Organisms

    i. Most common organisms include coagulase-negative staphylococci (i.e. *S. epidermidis*) and *Streptococcus* species.

    ii. Higher frequency of virulent organisms such as *Bacillus* species

        1. Severity is likely caused by enterotoxin-mediated reaction

    iii. Polymicrobial infection is more frequent following open-globe injuries, likely because they are part of the normal skin flora and regularly contaminate open wounds

        1. *Staphylococcus epidermidis*

        2. *Streptococcus* species

    iv. Fulminant endophthalmitis

        1. *Pseudomonas* species

        2. *Clostridium* species

    3. Suspect fungal in the setting of vegetable matter injuries such as tree branch or thorn injury

      a. *Candida, Aspergillus, Paecilomyces, Fusarium, Dematacious*

e. Management: No large randomized study showing benefit of therapy for traumatic endophthalmitis but guidelines are based on common practice.

    i. Repair of open globe as soon as possible

    ii. Intravitreal antibiotic injections as soon as possible

      1. Vancomycin 1 mg/0.1 mL or Clindamycin 500 mcg/0.1 mL and
      2. Ceftazidime 2.25 mg/0.1 mL or Amikacin 400 mcg/0.1 mL

    iii. Vitrectomy for post-traumatic endophthalmitis often recommended especially for fulminant cases before intravitreal antibiotic injection

    iv. Systemic antiobiotic (oral or intravenous) with good ocular penetration recommended

      1. Intravenous (IV) Vancomycin, Ceftazidime or
      2. Oral or IV Fluoroquinolone

f. Prognosis

    i. Better presenting visual acuity and shorter time from injury to presentation fosters a better prognosis

3. Macula-Sparing Traumatic Retinal Detachment

a. Background

    i. 29% of open globe injuries may have or develop a retinal detachment; however, may not appear until days to weeks after the initial traumatic event

    ii. Increased risk of retinal detachment associated with presence of a vitreous hemorrhage, higher zone of injury, and poor visual acuity at the time of presentation

    iii. No known studies comparing timing of surgery in the setting of trauma

    iv. Prompt surgery may be technically more difficult, with increased incidence of vitreoretinal adhesions particularly at the vitreous base and risk of bleeding. In comparison, delayed surgery (day 14) may allow for a posterior vitreous detachment and easier to cut vitreous

4. Open Globe Repair

Prompt repair of an open globe is standard of care. However, the following points are areas of controversy in the acute management of open globes involving the posterior segment

a. Role of vitrectomy in the acute setting beyond above indications
b. The ideal timing of vitrectomy after globe injury if indicated
c. The potential benefit of prophylactic cryotherapy for posterior laceration
d. The potential benefit of prophylactic scleral buckle
e. The use of prophylactic antibiotics use and route of administration
f. Vitrectomy versus vitreous tap for traumatic endophthalmitis
g. Concurrent intraocular lens implantation in the acute setting of a traumatic cataract

Indications for Non-urgent Vitreoretinal Surgical Intervention:

1. Macula-involving Traumatic Retinal Detachment (RD)

a. Refer to Chapter 24 on RD for details on surgical techniques.
b. Prognosis of RD following trauma

   i. Higher frequency of proliferative vitreo-retinopathy (PVR) in pediatric population because greater fibroblastic activity in children than in adults, higher percentage of vitreous hemorrhage, and delay in intervention

   ii. Poorer prognosis if undetermined or light perception or worse perioperative vision, or presence of PVR grade C or worse, total retinal detachment, and macula-off status

c. Ideal timing for surgery in RD repair in traumatic eyes

   i. Controversial

   ii. Proponents of vitrectomy between 4 and 10 days after injury, or before 2 weeks, argue that uveal congestion that develops after trauma may increase the risk of uncontrollable hemorrhage, and the lack of separation of the posterior vitreous makes complete removal difficult

   iii. Some argue that there is heightened fibrous proliferation when surgery is delayed by 2 weeks, which can inflict further retinal damage and increase the difficulties of surgery. Others argue that vitrectomy performed 14 days after penetrating ocular injury is associated with improved visual outcomes

d. Blunt versus penetrating trauma

    i.   Blunt injury can affect internal structures of the eye and similarly, optic nerve and extent of the wound can be posterior to recti insertion resulting in poorer final vision outcome

2. Suprachoroidal Detachment or Hemorrhage

a. Timing of surgery

    i.   Traditionally, surgery is delayed until after autolysis (or liquefaction) of the clot so that drainage is easier and more complete (approximately 7 to 10 days)

    ii.   Some argue that earlier intervention, with or without vitrectomy and intraocular gas, produces superior visual outcomes

    iii.   Follow liquefaction of clot via B-scan ultrasound to optimize the timing of surgical intervention

    iv.   Indications for surgical drainage include recalcitrant pain, increased intraocular pressure (e.g. from angle closure), retinal detachment, and apposition choroidal detachments in order to prevent secondary traction or rhegmatogenous retinal detachments. Surgical goals include separation of kissing choroidal detachments by one half of their original height

b. Medical Adjuncts

    i.   Topical therapy

        1. Cycloplegia with atropine

        2. Steroids with prednisolone acetate, or difluprednate Durezol)

    ii.   Oral therapy

        1. Medrol dose-pak (methylprednisolone) or prednisone 1 mg/kg/day if patient has pain and/or non-diabetic

c. Surgical Technique

    i.   Correct primary or secondary causes of choroidal detachment (e.g. hypotony from wound leak, shallow retinal detachment, or ciliary body detachment)

    ii.   Pressurize the eye from within, often with an anterior chamber maintainer/infusion line

iii. Make a full thickness scleral incision 5–8 mm posterior to the limbus in areas where the choroidal detachments are most prominent. Incisions are circumferential or radial and at least 2 mm in length

iv. The incisions are left open after surgery to encourage continued drainage of fluid during the post-operative period

v. Most frequent complication is an inability to achieve adequate drainage

d. Concurrent retinal detachment

i. Retinal detachment in an eye with concurrent choroidal detachment or hemorrhage in all four quadrants correlates with poor visual outcome

ii. Scleral buckling and long-term tamponade with silicone oil may be required given high risk of PVR

e. Prognosis

i. Residual choroidal hemorrhage after drainage usually resolves over a few weeks to months

ii. Eyes should be monitored for hypotony, retinal detachment, proliferative vitreoretinopathy, pain and phthisis

3. Non-clearing vitreous hemorrhage

a. Background

i. Marked vitreous hemorrhage is associated with poor visual prognosis in ocular trauma

ii. Presence of large amounts of blood in the vitreous cavity for long periods is associated with enhanced proliferative vitreoretinopathy, ghost-cell glaucoma and hemosiderosis bulbi

iii. Vitreous hemorrhage is an important factor for development of PVR which is the most common reason for eventual failure of RD surgery

iv. Timing of vitrectomy is controversial

1. Vitrectomy 2 months or longer after injury is associated with poor visual outcome and anatomical success

2. Some reports state there is no significant difference between timing of vitrectomy

4. Traumatic Cataract or Lens Subluxation

a. Background

    i. Injury is rarely limited to the lens alone and may be associated with injuries to the zonules, posterior capsule and posterior segment

    ii. May occur after blunt and penetrating eye injuries

b. Surgical Technique

    i. Anterior versus pars planar approach

    ii. Triamcinolone can be injected into the AC to assess the extent of the prolapsed vitreous

    iii. Intraocular lens (IOL) options

        1. Single piece lens in the bag if intact capsular bag

        2. If capsular support is lacking, consider

            a. IOL in the anterior chamber

            b. Iris-sutured IOL in the posterior chamber

            c. Sclera-fixated IOL in the posterior chamber

            d. Sutureless, fibrin glue-assisted lens in the posterior chamber

c. Timing of surgery: not urgent unless intraocular pressure or inflammation is not controlled with medical therapy

References

1. Shock JP, Adams D. Long-term visual acuity results after penetrating and perforating ocular injuries. *Am J Ophthalmol* 1985;100:714–8.
2. Lin KY, Ngai P, Echegoyen JC, *et al.* Imaging in orbital trauma. *Saudi J Ophthalmol* 2012;26:427–432.
3. Bai HQ, Yao L, Meng XX, *et al.* Visual outcome following intraocular foreign bodies: A retrospective review of 5-year clinical experience. *Eur J Ophthalmol* 2011;21: 98–103.
4. Azad RV, Kumar N, Sharma YR *et al.* Role of prophylactic scleral buckling in the management of retained intraocular foreign bodies. *Clin Exp Ophthalmol* 2004;32:58–61.
5. Al–Mezaine HS, Osman EA, Kangave D *et al.* Risk factors for culture-positive endophthalmitis after repair of open globe injuries. *Eur J Ophthalmol* 2010;20:201–208.
6. Brinton GS, Topping TM, Hyndiuk RA *et al.* Posttraumatic endophthalmitis. *Arch Ophthalmol* 1984;102:547–550.
7. Snell Jr AC. Perforating ocular injuries. *Am J Ophthalmol* 1945;28:263–281.
8. Ahmed Y, Schimel AM, Pathengay A, *et al.* Endophthalmitis following open-globe injuries. *Eye* 2012;26:212–217.
9. Boldt HC, Pulido JS, Blodi CF. Rural endophthalmitis. *Ophthalmol* 1989;96: 1722–1726.
10. Thompson JT, Parver LM, Enger CL *et al.* Infectious endophthalmitis after penetrating injuries with retained intraocular foreign bodies. *Ophthalmol* 1993;100:1468–1474.
11. Essex RW, Yi Q, Charles PG *et al.* Post-traumatic endophthalmitis. *Ophthalmol* 2004;111:2015–2022.
12. Al-Omran AM, Abboud EB, Abu El-Asrar AMA. Microbiologic spectrum and visual outcome of posttraumatic endophthalmitis. *Retina* 2007;27:236–42.
13. Bhagat N, Nagori S, Zarbin M. Post-traumatic infectious endophthalmitis. *Surv Ophthalmol* 2011;56:214–251.
14. Chhabra S, Kunimoto DY, Kazi L *et al.* Endophthalmitis after open globe injury: Microbiologic spectrum and susceptibilities of isolates. *Am J Ophthalmol* 2006;142:852–854.
15. Wykoff CC, Flynn Jr HW, Miller D *et al.* Exogenous fungal endophthalmitis: Microbiology and clinical outcomes. *Ophthalmol* 2008;115:1501–1507.
16. Stryjewski TP, Andreoli CM, Eliott D. Retinal detachment after open globe injury. *Ophthalmol* 2014;121:327–333.
17. Mittra RA, Mieler RF. Controversies in the management of open-globe injuries involving the posterior segment. *Surv Ophthalmol* 1999;44:215–225.
18. Wang NK, Chen YP, Yeung L, *et al.* Traumatic pediatric retinal detachment following open globe injury. *Ophthalmologica* 2007;221:255–263.
19. Cupples HP, Whitmore PV, Wertz FD III, *et al.* Ocular trauma treated by vitreous surgery. *Retina* 1983;3:103–107.

20. Ryan SJ, Allen AW. Pars plana vitrectomy in ocular trauma. *Am J Ophthalmol* 1979;88:483–491.
21. Conway BP, Michels RG. Vitrectomy techniques in the management of selected penetrating ocular injuries. *Ophthalmol* 1978;85:560–583.
22. Cleary PE, Ryan SJ. Vitrectomy in penetrating eye injury. Results of a controlled trial of vitrectomy in an experimental posterior penetrating eye injury in the rhesus monkey. *Arch Ophthalmol* 1981;99:287–292.
23. Hermsen V. Vitrectomy in severe ocular trauma. *Ophthalmologica* 1984;189:86–92.
24. Vatne HO, Syrdalen P. Vitrectomy in double perforating eye injuries. *Acta Ophthalmol* 1985;63:552–556.
25. WuDunn D, Ryser D, Cantor LB. Surgical drainage of choroidal effusions following glaucoma surgery. *J Glaucoma* 2005;14:103–108.
26. Reynolds MG, Haimovici R, Flynn HW, *et al.* Suprachoroidal hemorrhage. Clinical features and results of secondary surgical management. *Ophthalmol* 1993;100:460–465.
27. Brinton GS, Aaberg TM, Reeser FH, *et al.* Surgical results in ocular trauma involving the posterior segment. *Am J Ophthalmol* 1982;93:271–278.
28. Cardillo JA, Stout JT, LaBree L, *et al.* Post-traumatic proliferative vitreoretinopathy. The epidemiologic profile, onset, risk factors, and visual outcome. *Ophthalmol* 1997;104:1166–1173.
29. Spraul CW, Grossniklaus HE. Vitreous hemorrhage. *Surv Ophthalmol* 1997;42:3–39.
30. Vergara O, Ogden T, Ryan S. Posterior penetrating injury in the rabbit eye: Effect of blood and ferrous ions. *Exp Eye Res* 1989;49:1115–1126.
31. Miyake Y, Ando F. Surgical results of vitrectomy intraocular trauma. *Retina* 1983;3:265–268.
32. Ahmadieh H, Sohelian M, Sajjadi H, *et al.* Vitrectomy in ocular trauma. Factors influencing final visual outcomes. *Retina* 1993;13:107–113.
33. Chaundhry NA, Belfort A, Flynn HW Jr, *et al.* Combined lensectomy, vitrectomy, and scleral fixation of intraocular lens implant after closed-globe injury. *Ophthalmic Surg Lasers* 1999;30:375–381.
34. Agarwal A, Kumar DA, Jacob S, *et al.* Fibrin glue-assisted sutureless posterior chamber intraocular lens implantation in eyes with deficient posterior capsules. *J Cataract Refract Surg* 2008;34:1433–1438.

Chapter 23: Non-surgical Management of Posterior Segment Trauma

Eric K. Chin, David R.P. Almeida and Susanna S. Park

1. Traumatic Maculopathy/Commotio Retinae

a. Acute manifestations on OCT and fundus exam

   i. OCT findings

      1. Swelling of the outer retina, with preservation of the inner retinal structure including the foveal pit

      2. Disruption of the IS/OS photoreceptor junction, increased reflectivity, cell infiltration of the retinal wall and retinal pigment epithelium detachment

   ii. Fundus findings

      1. Whitening corresponds to photoreceptor outer segment disruption on histopathology

b. Chronic manifestations on OCT and fundus exam

   i. OCT may have variable level of disruption of photoreceptor reflectivity — See Figure 1

   ii. Permanent IS/OS injunction defects on OCT with reduced electroretinal activity are more likely to represent irreversible photoreceptor damage

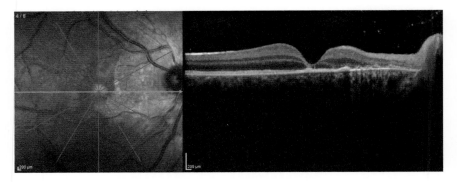

Figure 1. OCT image of chronic changes in the outer retina following *commotio retinae* between the fovea and optic nerve in the setting of acute blunt trauma.

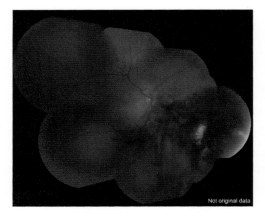

Figure 2. Sclopeteria following blunt trauma.

c. Visual prognosis

    i. May cause permanent loss of vision if fovea is damaged

    ii. Final visual acuity does not always correlate with the degree of retinal whitening at acute presentation

2. Traumatic Choroidal Rupture

a. Clinical features

    i. Acutely, the rupture site may be obscured by hemorrhage

ii. Yellow or white crescent-shaped subretinal streak on funduscopy concentric to disc or parallel to the ora serrata

iii. Traumatic optic neuropathy may also be present

b. Late complications

i. Risk of developing a choroidal neovascular membrane (CNVM)

3. Chorioretinitis Sclopetaria

a. Background

i. Fundus appearance after full-thickness break of the choroid and retina as result of a high-velocity missile striking or passing adjacent to, but not penetrating, the globe

b. Mechanism

i. Rapid deformation of the globe by a high-velocity object or its shock wave causes a sudden increase in the stress in the sclera, choroid, retina, and posterior vitreous cortex, without directly contacting the globe

ii. Rupture occurs in areas where induced tensile stretch/force is greater than the tensile strength of the tissue

iii. Accompanied by retraction of retina and choroid, and exposure of bare sclera

c. Clinical features — See Figure 2

i. Acute intraocular hemorrhages from rupture of choroid and retinal vessels by direct concussive forces of projectile

ii. Macular disruption may occur from indirect countercoup trauma generated by the concussive force of missile passing close to the globe

iii. Eventually blood is resorbed and the resultant defects are replaced by fibrous tissue

d. Prognosis

i. Visual acuity at presentation is related to the extent and location of the chorioretinal rupture

ii. Poor presenting visual acuity carries a worse visual prognosis for the patient

e. Management

    i. No effective treatment, and typically observation only

4. Purtscher's Retinopathy

a. Mechanism

    i. "Purtscher" by definition is associated with trauma

b. Differential diagnosis

    i. Pseudo-Purtscher retinopathy occurs with acute pancreatitis, malignant hypertension, collagen vascular disease (e.g. systemic lupus erythematosis, scleroderma, dermatomyositis, Sjogren syndrome), thrombotic thrombocytopenic purpura, chronic renal failure, amniotic fluid embolus, retrobulbar anesthesia, orbital steroid injection, alcohol usage and long bone fractures

c. Clinical course

    i. History of compression injury to the chest, head or lower extremities, but not a direct ocular injury

    ii. Decreased vision, often sudden and can be severe

    iii. Signs

        1. Changes are typically bilateral but may be asymmetric or unilateral

        2. Multiple patches of retinal whitening, large cotton-wool spots and hemorrhages that surround the optic disc following multiple long bone fractures with fat emboli or severe compressive injuries to the chest or head

        3. May have optic disc edema and a positive relative afferent defect

d. Prognosis

    i. Usually resolves over weeks to months

e. Treatment

    i. None needed

References

Pham TQ, Chua B, Gorbatov M, *et al*. Optical coherence tomography findings of acute traumatic maculopathy following motor vehicle accident. *Am J Ophthalmol* 2007;143:348–350.

Mendes S, Campos A, Beselga D, *et al*. Traumatic maculopathy six months after injury: A clinical case report. *Case Rep Ophthalmol* 2014;5:78–82.

Mansour AM, Green WR, Hogge C. Histopathology of commotio retinae. *Retina* 1992;12:24–28.

Saleh M, Letsch J, Bourcier T, *et al*. Long-term outcomes of acute traumatic maculopathy. *Retina* 2011;31:2037–2043.

Richards RD, West CE, Meisels AA. Chorioretinitis sclopetaria. *Am J Ophthalmol* 1968;66:852–860.

Papakostas TD, Yonekawa Y, Skondra D, *et al*. Traumatic chorioretinal rupture (sclopetaria). *Int Ophthalmol Clin* 2013;54:119–125.

Martin DF, Awh CC, McCuen BW 2nd, *et al*. Treatment and pathogenesis of traumatic chorioretinal rupture (sclopetaria). *Am J Ophthalmol* 1994;117:190–200.

SECTION 7: RETINAL DETACHMENT

Chapter 24: Retinal Detachment and Proliferative Vitreoretinopathy

Glenn Yiu

Risk Factors

1. History of Retinal detachment (RD) in fellow eye (10–15%)
2. Myopia/long axial length (7–8%)
3. Lattice Degeneration (1%)
4. Family History of retinal detachment
5. Male gender

Etiology

1. Retinal tear with Posterior vitreous detachment (PVD)

    a. Incidence of PVD (> age 70): 63%
    b. Incidence of retinal tear after symptomatic PVD: 10–15%
    c. Incidence of retinal tear after hemorrhagic PVD: 50–70%
    d. Incidence of retinal tear after non-hemorrhagic PVD: 2–4%

2. Atrophic hole in lattice degeneration

    a. Incidence of lattice degeneration: 6–10%
    b. Incidence of lattice degeneration in RD: 20–30%

3. Retinal dialysis

    a. Avulsion of vitreous base
    b. Commonly occurs after blunt trauma
    c. Most common locations inferotemporal and superonasal

Differential Diagnosis

1. Tractional Retinal Detachment

    a. Pre-retinal traction causing detachment
    b. May occur along with rhegmatogenous RD
    c. Causes:

        i. Proliferative diabetic retinopathy (PDR)
        ii. Retinopathy of prematurity (ROP)
        iii. Familial exudative vitreoretinopathy (FEVR)
        iv. Toxocariasis
        v. Sickle Cell Retinopathy
        vi. Post-trauma

2. Serous Retinal Detachment

    a. Serous fluid with no retinal break
    b. Fluid may be turbid and shifts to dependent position
    c. Causes

        i. Neovascular Age-Related Macular Degeneration (AMD)
        ii. Polypoidal choroidal vasculopathy
        iii. Central serous chorioretinopathy
        iv. Optic nerve pit
        v. Vogt–Koyanagi–Harada (VKH) syndrome
        vi. Sympathetic ophthalmia
        vii. Posterior scleritis
        viii. Hyoptony
        ix. Severe hypertension/pre-eclampsia
        x. Choroidal or retinal tumor, benign and neoplastic
        xi. Coat's disease and other retinal vasculopathies
        xii. Infections (e.g. toxoplasmosis, syphilis)
            (MIGHT GROUP V–VII, XII under Uveitis, usually VKH and Post scleritis)

3. Degenerative Retinoschisis

    a. Splitting of retina at outer plexiform layer ("old person's layer")
    b. Smooth, dome-shaped; usually inferotemporal
    c. May have inner retinal break; becomes RD if outer retinal break occurs
    d. Distinguish from RD (See Table 1)

Table 1. How To Distinguish Degenerative Retinoschisis from Retinal Detachment

	Degenerative Retinoschisis	**Retinal Detachment**
Scotoma	Absolute	Relative
Vitreous pigment or blood	Rare	Common
Appearance	Smooth, dome-shaped	Corrugated, irregular surface
Pigment line if chronic	None	Present
Response to laser	Blanches	Does not blanch

Initial Evaluation: History

1. Location and Type of visual loss

    a. Typically flashes or floaters preceding a curtain or veil obscuring vision
    b. If visual loss respects horizontal meridian, suspect optic nerve etiology
    c. If visual loss respects vertical meridian, suspect neurological etiology
    d. Ocular pain or discomfort rare, unless other ocular pathology (e.g. ocular surface disease, uveitis) also present

2. Onset/duration of symptoms

    a. Visual Prognosis is better if repaired within 7–10 days of symptom onset for macular involving RD
    b. If asymptomatic, look for pigment demarcation line to suggest chronicity (Figure 1); may observe if not threatening macula

3. Past ocular/surgical history

    a. Any history of RD, high myopia, lattice degeneration, etc.
    b. Any recent ocular surgery or laser (YAG capsulotomy)

4. Other considerations

    a. Other health problems — may affect type of anesthesia; avoid Scleral Buckle (SB) for patients with sickle cell disease due to risk for anterior segment ischemia
    b. Blood thinner use — may avoid SB or retrobulbar anesthesia
    c. Ability to position — may determine suitability for gas tamponade
    d. Anticipated air travel — may determine suitability for gas tamponade

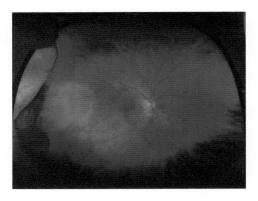

Figure 1. Chronic retinal detachment with demarcation line in the temporal periphery.

Initial Evaluation: Exam

1. Size and location of RD

   a. Status of macula/fovea — determines urgency for repair
   b. If chronic or pigment demarcation line present — consider observation if asymptomatic

2. Size, location, and number of retinal breaks

   a. Use Lincoff rules to help identify breaks (see Figure 2)

      i. In superior, temporal, or nasal RDs, the etiologic break is within 1.5 clock hours of the superior border of RD
      ii. In total or superior RD that crosses the 12 o'clock meridian, the etiologic break is within 1.5 clock hours to either side of 12 o'clock
      iii. In inferior nonbullous RDs, the etiologic break is on the side of the optic disc with the higher border
      iv. In inferior bullous RDs, the etiologic break is usually superior near 12 o'clock

   b. If no breaks identified, consider SB and/or pars plana vitrectomy (PPV)

      i. Detailed intraoperative examination may allow breaks to be identified.

   c. If no breaks identified and RD is inferior, rule out serous RD

Rules to Find the Primary Break

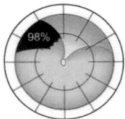

Rule 1:

Superior temporal or nasal detachments:
In 98%, the primary break lies within 1$\frac{1}{2}$ clock-hours of the highest border.

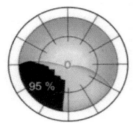

Rule 2:

Total or superior detachments that cross the 12 o'clock meridian:
In 93%, the primary break is at 12 o'clock or in a triangle, the apex of which is at the ora serrata, and the sides of which extend 1$\frac{1}{2}$ clock-hours to either side of 12 o'clock.

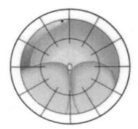

Rule 3:

Inferior detachments:
In 95%, the higher side of the detachment indicates on which side of the disc an inferior break lies.

Rule 4:

"Inferior" bullous detachment:
Inferior bullae in a rhegmatogenous detachment originate from a superior break.

Figure 2. Lincoff rules for finding a retinal break.

3. Presence of PVD

   a. If PVD absent or incomplete, avoid pneumatic retinopexy; consider PPV and/or SB
   b. If PVD present, consider pneumatic retinopexy, PPV and/or SB

4. Lens status

   a. If phakic, consider pneumatic retinopexy or SB first, then consider PPV
   b. If pseudophakic, consider pneumatic retinopexy, PPV and/or SB

5. Presence of other ocular pathology

   a. Lattice Degeneration — consider SB or PPV with prophylactic laser
   b. Proliferative Vitreoretinopathy (PVR) — consider PPV (concurrent SB for more advanced cases)

      i. Grade A: vitreous haze or pigment clumps
      ii. Grade B: retinal wrinkling/stiffness, vessel tortuosity, rolled/irregular edge of break, decreased vitreous mobility
      iii. Grade C: focal, diffuse, or circumferential full-thickness folds, subretinal strands
      (A = anterior to equator; P = posterior to equator)

      1. Type 1 (P): focal (starfold)
      2. Type 2 (P): diffuse
      3. Type 3 (A/P): subretinal
      4. Type 4 (A): circumferential
      5. Type 5 (A): anterior displacement

   c. Media opacity (e.g. vitreous hemorrhage, corneal opacity) — consider PPV

MANAGEMENT*

Note: The management of retinal detachment is complex and varied. The recommendations presented in this section reflects only the opinion of the authors, and does not constitute the standard of care in all cases

1. Principles of RD repair

   a. Identify all retinal breaks and traction
   b. Approximate detached retina to the retinal pigment epithelium (RPE)
   c. Relieve all vitreoretinal traction (SB or PPV)
   d. Seal all retinal breaks by creating a chorioretinal adhesion (laser or cryotherapy)

Table 2. Advantages & Disadvantages of Retinal Detachment Repair Methods

	Advantages	**Disadvantages**
Pneumatic Retinopexy	Office procedure Low cost Less patient discomfort Fast visual recovery No diplopia No induced astigmatism or refractive changes	Requires strict positioning Not effective for inferior breaks Not effective for PVR Less effective for lattice Lower rates of primary success Does not relieve traction
Scleral Buckle	Can treat all primary RD Reduces vitreous traction Less cataract formation than PPV Prophylaxis against future PVR	Change in refractive error More patient discomfort Risk of diplopia/strabismus Risk of infection/buckle extrusion/subretinal bleeding
Pars Plana Vitrectomy	Can treat primary and recurrent RD Can relieve PVR and traction Less patient discomfort Intraoperative reattachment Improved peripheral visualization	High cost of instruments High rates of cataract formation Requires head positioning Slight risk of endophthalmitis

2. Pneumatic Retinopexy

    a. Office-based intravitreal injection of air or gas to tamponade retinal break, followed by creation of chorioretinal adhesion by cryotherapy (same day) or laser (1–2 days later)

    b. Ideal for

       i. Primary RD with single retinal break in superior 8 clock hours

       ii. Contraindications to anesthesia or surgery

       iii. Residual superior radial folds with subretinal fluid after SB surgery

    c. Criteria

       i. Good visualization of peripheral retina and break

       ii. Single/multiple breaks each <1 clock hour, spanning <3 clock hours in superior 8 clock hours

       iii. No PVR or extensive lattice degeneration

       iv. Ability to maintain head position

d.   Gas choice

   i.   Buoyant force pushes retina against the RPE
   ii.   Surface Tension prevents gas from passing through tear
   iii.   Characteristics of gas (see Table 3)
   iv.   Arc of contact (see Table 4)

e.   Complications

   i.   Elevated intraocular pressure:

     1.   Monitor for central retinal artery perfusion after gas injection
     2.   Consider paracentesis prior to gas injection in patients with glaucoma
     3.   Avoid N_2O for general anesthesia (tissue nitrogen enters gas bubble)
     4.   Avoid air travel and driving to higher altitudes while gas is present
     5.

   ii.   "Fish Eggs"

     1.   If "Fish Eggs" occur, position bubbles away from retinal tear for 24 hours until bubbles coalesce, then resume proper position to minimize risk of subretinal gas (rare event even with Fish Eggs)

Table 3.   Characteristics of Gas Tamponade Agents.

Type	Expansion	Duration	Non-expansile Concentration
Air	0	4–7 days	—
SF6	2 times	14 days	25–30%
C2F6	3 times	35 days	20–25%
C3F8	4 times	60 days	15–16%

Table 4.   Geometry of Intraocular Gas Bubble.

Arc of bubble contact	Vitreous diameter 21 mm	Vitreous diameter 24 mm
90 degrees	0.28 mL	0.42 mL
120 degrees	0.75 mL	1.13 mL
150 degrees	1.49 mL	2.24 mL
180 degrees	2.40 mL	3.62 mL

    iii. Subretinal Gas

        1. For small amount of subretinal gas, scleral depression may be used to maneuver the bubble back into the vitreous cavity

        2. For large amount of subretinal gas, a needle may be required to vent the gas from the subretinal space

  f. Prognosis (based on multicenter trial comparing pneumatic retionpexy with for RD repair[7]):

    i. Primary reattachment: 73% (versus 82% after SB)

    ii. Final reattachment (after re-operation) 99% (versus 98% after SB)

    iii. Visual outcome >20/50: 88% (versus 69% after SB)

3. Scleral Buckling

  a. Indentation of eye wall with an external element to support the retinal break(s) and relieve vitreous traction

  b. Ideal for

    i. Primary RD in phakic eye

    ii. Young patients with attached/adherent posterior hyaloid

    iii. Retinal dialysis without retinal tear

  c. Criteria

    i. Good visualization of peripheral retina

    ii. No to minimal PVR

    iii. Not very posterior retinal tear(s): anterior to equator

  d. Band choice

    i. Types

      1. Encircling

        a. Good for multiple breaks along circumference, or if additional breaks are suspected along circumference

        b. Prophylaxis against PVR or additional breaks in the future

        c. May accommodate tires to support longer breaks

      2. Segmental /Circumferential

        a. Good for multiple breaks along circumference

        b. Preserves conjunctivae in uninvolved quadrants (e.g. for glaucoma tube)

   3. Segmental/Radial

     a. Good for radial breaks that extend more posteriorly
     b. More difficult to place

  ii. Shape & Size

     1. Shape and size of band must accommodate the dimensions of the retinal breaks
     2. Scleral arc length is longer than the chord length, when measured with calipers
     3. Vitreous cavity volume displacement: (See Table 5)

d. Band Placement

  i. Location

     1. The retinal breaks that are most posterior should be positioned on the posterior crest of the band

  ii. Height

     1. Adjust buckle element by 2 *pi* (6.28 mm) to increase buckle height by 1 mm
     2. Beware of "fish mouth" phenomenon resulting from radial folds with a highly-placed encircling band

e. Drainage

  i. Ideal for

     1. Highly bullous RD/inability to apply cryotherapy to detached retina
     2. Also allows intravitreal space for intravitreal air or gas injection

Table 5. Estimated Vitreous Cavity Volume Displacement of Scleral Buckles.

Scleral Buckle	Vitreous Cavity Volume Displacement
Half of 5 mm sponge	0.09–0.15 mL
3 × 5 mm sponge	0.11–0.20 mL
5 mm round sponge	0.14–0.22 mL
#240 style band	0.47–0.48 mL
#276 style band	1.08–1.13 mL
#287 style band	1.32–1.57 mL
#280 style band	1.82–1.88 mL

ii. Optimal location

1. In area of largest fluid collection
2. Above or below horizontal meridian; preferably nasal
3. Avoid large retinal breaks/run-through of vitreous
4. Under band if possible

iii. Complications

1. Retinal hole (rare)
2. Retinal incarceration (1–2%)
3. Subretinal hemorrhage (3–4%)

f. Post-operative complications

i. Recurrent retinal detachment

1. May occur due to inadequate buckle height, misplaced buckle position, missed retinal break, or "fish mouth" effect

ii. Band exposure, extrusion, or infection

1. Exposed bands are often colonized with micro-organisms even in the absence of a frank infection
2. Explantation is usually preferred over conjunctival revision due to the risk of creating a nidus for infection

iii. Band migration

1. Usually observed unless there is significant discomfort or diplopia

iv. Change in Refraction

1. Occurs due to change in geometry with scleral indentation
2. Patients should be cautioned about the likelihood of a myopic shift
3. Mean change: 1.5 diopters (check reference to confirm)

v. Diplopia

1. Usually occurs postoperatively and often improves with time
2. Consider explantation only if persistent and unable to manage with prisms alone

vi. Anterior segment ischemia

    1. Related to very high encircling bands and/or rectus muscle disinsertion

    2. Higher risk in sickle cell patient

    3. May present with corneal edema, pain, anterior chamber cell or flare

vii. Posterior cryotherapy

    1. Occurs due to inadvertent shaft indentation of retinal break

    2. Avoid by starting scleral depression more anteriorly

g. Prognosis (based on multicenter Scleral Buckle versus Vitrectomy study for RD repair):

    i. In phakic eyes: visual acuity change greater in SB group (-0.71 logMAR) than PPV group (-0.56 logMAR) ($P = 0.0005$); anatomic success similar between SB group (63.2%) and PPV group (62.8%) ($P = 0.9709$)

    ii. In pseudophakic eyes: visual acuity change similar between SB group (-0.56 logMAR) and PPV group (-0.64 logMAR) ($P = 0.09$); anatomic success greater in PPV group (72.0%) than SB group (53.4%) ($P = 0.0020$)

    iii. Cataract progression in phakic eyes is greater in PPV group (77.3%) than SB group (45.9%) ($P < 0.00005$)

4. Pars Plana Vitrectomy

a. Microsurgical removal of vitreous gel from the eye to relieve traction

b. Ideal for

    i. RD with multiple retinal breaks at different distances from the ora

    ii. RD with posterior retinal breaks

    iii. RD with extensive PVR

    iv. RD with significant media opacity

c. Visualization

    i. Lenses

        1. Contact lenses: eliminates all corneal asphericity; requires stabilization; less problems with fogging

        2. Non-contact lenses: hands-free operation; reduced lateral and axial resolution; fogging with moisture

   ii. Illumination

      1. Light pipe: produces focal, specular, or retro illumination; higher risk of phototoxicity if too close to retina
      2. Chandelier: produces diffuse illumination; allows bimanual manipulation
      3. Infusion chandelier: allows bimanual manipulation without additional port placement

  iii. Other tools

      1. Iris hooks — used for posterior synechiae or poor pharmacological dilation
      2. Corneal scraping — useful for corneal epithelial edema, especially in long cases
      3. Viscoelastic — used to remove IOL fogging, especially during fluid-air exchange in a pseudophakic eye without an intact posterior lens capsule (worse with silicone than acrylic or PMMA lenses)
      4. Temporary keratoprosthesis — used for eyes with corneal opacity requiring a penetrating keratoplasty or permanent keratoprosthesis
      5. Endoscopy — used for eyes with corneal opacity that is likely transient and does not require a permanent corneal transplantation

  iv. Adjunctive Reagents

      1. Triamcinolone — may be used to highlight vitreous gel or epiretinal membrane
      2. Indocyanine Green — may be used to stain the internal limiting membrane; does not stain epiretinal membranes

d. Modes

   i. Core vitrectomy

      1. "3D"— decreased cut rate with increased vacuum
      2. "Proportional vacuum"— constant cut rate with variable vacuum

  ii. Shave vitrectomy

      1. Close bias duty cycle (versus open bias duty cycle common in core vitrectomy)
      2. May employ higher or similar cut rate as core vitrectomy

    iii. Extrusion

        1. Aspiration without vitreous cutting
        2. Usually used for removal of blood or small debris, creation of drainage retinotomy, removal of subretinal fluid or blood, as well as fluid-fluid, fluid-air, or fluid-gas exchanges

    iv. Viscous fluid injection/extraction

        1. Usually used for silicone oil injection or removal
        2. May also be used for direct perfluorocarbon — silicone oil exchange

  e. Tamponades

    i. Gas

        1. Relatively inert; gradually reabsorbed into bloodstream
        2. At least 30cc required for complete equilibration of gas concentration
        3. See Tables 3 and 4
        4. Complications

            a. Elevated IOP — may result from incorrect concentration of gas, air travel, N2O anesthesia, or history of glaucoma
            b. Subretinal gas — often due to small gas bubbles; self-resolves

    ii. Perfluorocarbon (PFC)

        1. Intraoperative use only; permanent retinal changes if left for >2 weeks
        2. Ideal for: PVR, giant retinal tears, ocular trauma
        3. Uses

            a. Flattens RD without drainage retinotomy
            b. Opens fixed retinal folds

Table 6. Comparison of Tamponades

	Gas	**Perfluorocarbon**	**Silicone Oil**
Tamponade force	++++	++	+
Surface Tension	++++	++	++
Viscosity	−	+	+++

Table 7. Comparison of Types of Perfluorocarbon

	'Perfluoro-octane	Perfluoro-decalin	Perfluoro-phenanthrene
Specific Gravity	1.76	1.9	2.01
Refractive Index	1.27	1.31	1.33
Viscosity (cs)	0.8	2.7	8.0

    c. Displaces subretinal fluid or blood, or suprachoroidal hemorrhage

    d. Stabilizes macula for peripheral vitrectomy

    e. Floats lens fragments, intraocular lens, or foreign bodies

4. Types (See Table 7)

5. Post-operative complications

    a. Retained PFC

        i. May be intravitreal or subretinal (Figure 3)

        ii. Occurs more frequently after small gauge PPV

        iii. Observe if small bubble and peripheral location, but may migrate posteriorly

        iv. If subretinal, may be removed by direct aspiration using 39- or 41-gauge cannula or displacement with gas

        v. Performing a saline rinse after PFC removal intraoperatively may reduce the risk of PFC retention

iii. Silicone oil

1. Temporary or permanent replacement of vitreous gel

2. Not absorbed; must be removed surgically

3. Improved early visual recovery after surgery when compared to gas

4. Viscosity related to chain length of polymer

5. Indications:

    a. RD with PVR

    b. Giant retinal tears

    c. Complex pediatric RD

    d. Viral retinitis

    e. Trauma or Endophthalmitis

    f. RD associated with choroidal colobomas

    g. Monocular patient needing early visual recovery

6. Post-operative complications

   a. Change in refractive power   '

      i. Hyperopic shift in phakic or pseudophakic eyes due to increased index of refraction

      ii. Myopic shift in aphakic eyes due to formation of oil meniscus in the pupillary plane

   b. Anterior chamber silicone oil migration

      i. Occurs in aphakic or pseudophakic eyes where the lens-iris diaphragm may be compromised

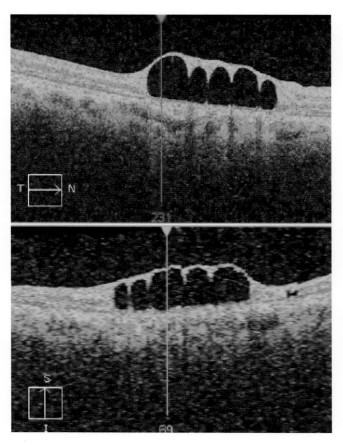

Figure 3. OCT showing retained subretinal perfluorocarbon.

      ii. Signs include posterior bulging iris, shimmering reflex on iris, absence of anterior chamber flare

      iii. Management includes inferior peripheral iridotomy, face down positioning, and injection of viscoelastic into the anterior chamber if the oil bubble is small

      iv. Silicone oil retention sutures may be used in aniridic eyes[10]

c. Glaucoma

      i. May be related to pupillary block, oil overfill, anterior chamber oil migration, or secondary open- or closed-angle glaucoma

      ii. Management includes topical or oral anti-hypertensives, creating or re-opening a peripheral iridotomy with laser or surgery, glaucoma drainage device, and/or silicone oil removal

      iii. Ensure IOP is normalized at the end of surgery to prevent silicone oil overfill

d. Keratopathy

      i. Results from silicone oil contact with corneal endothelium

      ii. Risk factors: preoperative pseudophakia or aphakia, iris neovascularization, postoperative aqueous flare, and need for reoperation

      iii. Prevent keratopathy by preventing silicone oil migration to anterior chamber

e. Emulsification

      i. Dispersion of large silicone oil bubble(s) into smaller droplets

      ii. Occurs due to shear forces from ocular movement

      iii. Likelihood of emulsification inversely proportional to viscosity

      iv. Ease of removal also inversely proportional to viscosity

      v. Emulsified droplets remain often after silicone oil removal

      vi. Multiple air-fluid exchange may reduce the risk of residual emulsified silicone oil droplets

      f.   Adhesion to Silicone IOL

          i.   Rarely occurs today due to decreased popularity of silicone IOL

   7. Prognosis (based on multicenter Silicone Study comparing silicone oil with gas for RD repair)

      a. No difference in rate of re-attachments, visual acuity, or glaucoma between silicone oil and C3F8 or SF6 gas

f.   Instruments

    i. Infusion cannula — place at an oblique angle to increase length of scleral tunnel; avoid excessively steep angle which may result in subretinal or suprachoroidal infusion

    ii. Forceps — used for various manipulations, including peeling of membranes

    iii. Pick — may be used to initiate membrane peel or aid with PVR dissection

    iv. Scraper — may be used to initiate membrane peel or disrupt fine membranes

    v. Scissors — useful for segmentation or delamination of tractional tissues

    vi. Endodiathermy — used to achieve hemostasis, mark retinal breaks, or prepare for retinotomy or retinectomy

    vii. Soft-tip cannula — useful for fluid-air or fluid-gas exchanges, aspiration of blood of subretinal fluid, and injection or removal of perfluorocarbon (not silicone oil)

    viii. Subretinal cannula — 39 or 41 gauge; useful for injection of fluid into subretinal space

h.   Post-operative complications

    i. Cataract

      1. Usually presents as nuclear sclerosis occurring within 12–24 months of PPV

      2. Hypothesized to result from the increased partial pressure of oxygen in the vitreous cavity after PPV

    ii. Wound leak

        1. minimize by suturing wounds, especially in cases with silicone oil

  i. Prognosis (based on multicenter SPR study comparing PPV with SB for RD repair)

Special Considerations

1. Proliferative Vitreoretinopathy (PVR)

    a. Phakic eyes with PVR detachments should have the crystalline lens removed

    b. Proliferative membrane mature between 4 and 8 weeks and becomes easier to peel but more extensive after that time period

    c. Retinotomy and retinectomy may be additionally required to relieve traction if the retinal fails to flatten after extensive removal of preretinal and subretinal membranes

    d. Perfluorocarbons may be used to stabilize the posterior retina when anterior membrane peeling or shaving of peripheral vitreous is performed

    e. Subretinal membranes do not always require removal, if not contributing to RD

    f. Scleral buckle may be used along with vitrectomy for prophylaxis against further PVR, unless extensive peripheral retinectomy is planned

    g. Silicone oil provides tamponade over a longer period of time to prevent re-detachment

    h. Small gauge instruments may experience flex when working extensively in the periphery

2. Giant Retinal Tear

    a. Circumferential retinal tear >90 degrees (Figure 4)

    b. PFC helps to flatten retina, but care must be taken to prevent slippage; may consider direct PFC– + silicone oil exchange

    c. If using SB, a broad, low band is recommended

    d. Prognosis: 51–79% primary reattachment; 79–94% final reattachment[12–14]

3. High Myopia

   a. In eyes with very long axial length, specialized instruments may be necessary or trocars may need to be removed to reach the posterior pole
   b. Scleral buckling may worsen the condition in some cases
   c. Macular buckling may be considered in select cases

4. Macular Hole

   a. In RDs involving a macular hole, the macular hole may not be the etiologic break resulting in the detachment
   b. Gas tamponade is usually recommended; ILM peeling may be helpful but difficult to perform

5. Subretinal Hemorrhage (SRH)

   a. Occurs commonly in neovascular AMD eyes in patients on anti-coagulation
   b. Size

       i. Small — less than 2 disc areas
       ii. Medium — greater than 2 disc areas up to vascular arcades
       iii. Large — extending past vascular arcades

   c. Management

       i. Observation with continued intravitreal anti-VEGF therapy for small or medium SRH

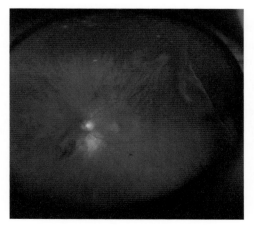

Figure 4. Retinal detachment with giant retinal tear. Pigment scarring from prior laser retinopexy can be seen inferonasally.

    ii. Pneumatic displacement with or without intravitreal Tissue plasminogen activator (TPA)

    iii. Pars plana vitrectomy with gas tamponade with or without subretinal TPA

6. Trauma (Refer to the section on Trauma for more details)

    a. Zones: higher zone denotes worse prognosis

        i. Zone I — cornea (including limbus)
        ii. Zone II — sclera between limbus and muscle insertions
        iii. Zone III — sclera posterior to muscle insertions

    b. Types: rupture has worse prognosis than laceration

        i. Rupture — following blunt eye injury; usually at equator behind muscle insertions
        ii. Laceration — penetrating injury by sharp object or projectile; may be penetrating (entry wound, but no exit wound) or perforating (entry and exit wounds)

    c. Intraocular foreign body (IOFB)

        i. Always ensure imaging studying performed to rule out IOFB
        ii. Increased incidence of endophthalmitis (7–13% in IOFB versus 2–8% in open globe injuries)
        iii. If IOFB present, emergent removal is usually necessary, except possibly high speed projectiles
        iv. Removal of IOFB may require foreign body forceps, or if ferromagnetic, an intraocular or external magnet

    d. Management

        i. PPV for trauma should be performed 7–14 day after injury
        ii. Prophylactic scleral buckle may be considered for Zone III injuries to prevent secondary retinal detachment

7. Keratoprosthesis (K-pro)

    a. Without a visible limbus, trocars for PPV should be placed 9 mm from the center of the K-pro

    b. Contact wide-angle lenses provide superior visualization through the K-pro optic

    c. Care should be taken due to poor visualization of the peripheral retina

References

1. WE Benson. Retinal Detachment: Diagnosis and Management. Philadelphia: Harper & Row Publishers Inc.
2. Hassan TS, Sarrafizadeh R, Ruby AJ, *et al.* The effect of duration of macular detachment on results after the scleral buckle repair of primary, macula-off retinal detachments. *Ophthalmol* 2002;109:146–152.
3. Diederen RM, La Heij EC, Kessels AG. Scleral buckling surgery after macula-off retinal detachment: worse visual outcome after more than 6 days. *Ophthalmol* 2007;114:705–709.
4. Kim JD, Pham HH, Lai MM, *et al.* Effect of symptom duration on outcomes following vitrectomy repair of primary macula-off retinal detachments. *Retina* 2013;33:1931–1937.
5. Ross WH, Kozy DW. Visual recovery in macula-off rhegmatogenous retinal detachments. *Ophthalmol* 1998;105:2149–2153.
6. Brod RD, Flynn HW, Jr., Lightman DA. Asymptomatic rhegmatogenous retinal detachments. *Arch Ophthalmol* 1995;113:1030–1032.
7. Tornambe PE, Hilton GF. Pneumatic retinopexy. A multicenter randomized controlled clinical trial comparing pneumatic retinopexy with scleral buckling. The Retinal Detachment Study Group. *Ophthalmol* 1989;96:772–783; discussion 784.
8. Heimann H, Bartz-Schmidt KU, Bornfeld N, *et al.* Scleral buckling versus primary vitrectomy in rhegmatogenous retinal detachment: A prospective randomized multicenter clinical study. *Ophthalmol* 2007;114:2142–2154.
9. Garg SJ, Theventhiran AB. Retained subretinal perfluorocarbon liquid in microincision 23-gauge versus traditional 20-gauge vitrectomy for retinal detachment repair. *Retina* 2012;32:2127–2132.
10. Gentile RC, Eliott D. Silicone oil retention sutures in aphakic eyes with iris loss. *Arch Ophthalmol* 2010;128:1596–1599.
11. Abrams GW, Azen SP, McCuen BW, 2nd, *et al.* Vitrectomy with silicone oil or long-acting gas in eyes with severe proliferative vitreoretinopathy: Results of additional and long-term follow-up. Silicone Study Report 11. *Arch Ophthalmol* 1997;115:335–344.
12. Kertes PJ, Wafapoor H, Peyman GA, *et al.* The management of giant retinal tears using perfluoroperhydrophenanthrene. A multicenter case series. Vitreon collaborative study group. *Ophthalmol* 1997;104:1159–1165.
13. Scott IU, Murray TG, Flynn HW, Jr, *et al.* Perfluoron Study G. Outcomes and complications associated with giant retinal tear management using perfluoro-n-octane. *Ophthalmol* 2002;109:1828–1833.
14. Al-Khairi AM, Al-Kahtani E, Kangave D, *et al.* Prognostic factors associated with outcomes after giant retinal tear management using perfluorocarbon liquids. *Eur J Ophthalmol* 2008;18:270–277.
15. Yiu G, Mahmoud TH. Subretinal hemorrhage. *Dev Ophthalmol* 2014;54:213–222.

16. Kuhn F, Maisiak R, Mann L, *et al.* The Ocular Trauma Score (OTS). *Ophthalmol Clin North Am* 2002;15:163–165, vi.

17. Colyer MH, Weber ED, Weichel ED, *et al.* Delayed intraocular foreign body removal without endophthalmitis during operations iraqi freedom and enduring freedom. *Ophthalmol* 2007;114:1439–1447.

18. Stone TW, Siddiqui N, Arroyo JG, *et al.* Primary scleral buckling in open-globe injury involving the posterior segment. *Ophthalmol* 2000;107:1923–1926.

19. Arroyo JG, Postel EA, Stone T, *et al.* A matched study of primary scleral buckle placement during repair of posterior segment open globe injuries. *Br J Ophthalmol* 2003;87:75–78.

SECTION 8: ONCOLOGY

Chapter 25: Current Treatment Options for Intraocular Retinoblastoma

Jonathan W. Kim

1. Retinoblastoma Epidemiology

— Incidence: 1/20,000 live births
— Survival: 95–99% in U.S. and Europe

2. Overall Treatment Approaches

A. 1960's: external radiation therapy for better eye, enucleation for advanced eye
B. 1995–2008: systemic chemotherapy combined with focal modalities
C. 2008–2014: emergence of local or regional therapies (e.g. intra-arterial chemotherapy and intravitreal injection)

3. Classification System (Grouping)

International Classification of Intraocular Retinoblastoma predicts success with chemoreduction protocols

Group A. Small tumors <3 mm in diameter (Figure 1)

   a. 90–100% success rate with focal modalities (i.e. photocoagulation and cryotherapy).

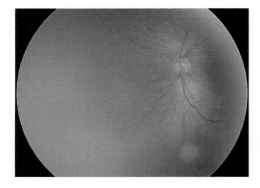

Figure 1. Fundus photograph of Group A retinoblastoma. This RETCAM wide-angle fundus photograph of the left eye of this one-year old boy shows a single white retinal lesion in the inferior mid-periphery measuring about 2 mm in diameter. (Courtesy of Susanna S. Park)

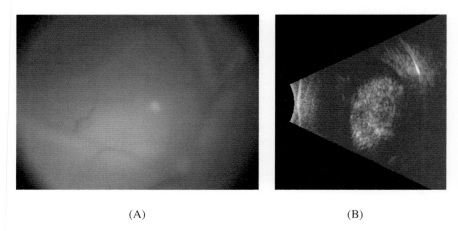

(A)   (B)

Figure 2. Group E Retinoblastoma. (A) RETCAM wide-angle fundus photograph of the right eye of the patient in Fig. 1 show a total bullous retinal elevation with tumor seeding. (B) B-scan ultrasound image of the eye shows a large posterior segment mass filling >50% of the globe with marked shadowing with tumor calcification. This eye was enucleated and histopathology showed retinoblastoma with high risk features, i.e. invasion of tumor into the choroid. The patient underwent systemic chemotherapy. (Figure courtesy of Susanna S. Park)

Group B. Tumors >3 mm in diameter or <3 mm from fovea or <1.5 mm from optic disc (up to 6 mm of subretinal fluid)

    b. 90–100% success rate with chemoreduction protocols

        i. 3 cycles of chemotherapy combined with focal consolidation

    c. brachytherapy is an option if peripheral and unilateral

Group C. Tumors with localized vitreous or subretinal seeding <3 mm from margin

    a. 80–90% success rate with chemoreduction protocols

        i. 3–6 cycles of chemotherapy + focal modalities

    b. brachytherapy is an option if peripheral and unilateral

Group D. Tumors with subretinal or vitreous seeding >3 mm from margin or >1 quadrant of subretinal fluid

    c. 47% success rate with chemoreduction protocols
    d. enucleation if unilateral and poor visual potential
    e. unilateral with visual potential: six cycles of chemoreduction or intra-arterial chemotherapy
    f. bilateral with Group D (at least one eye): 6 cycles of chemoreduction

Group E. Eyes with large tumors fulfiling following criteria:

    a. Neovascular glaucoma (high IOP)
    b. Vitreous hemorrhage obscuring view
    c. Tumor extending anterior to vitreous face (touching lens)
    d. Tumor mass filling more than half of posterior segment (Figure 2)
    e. Treatment for Group E is enucleation
    f. 24% risk of high risk histopathologic features

4. Systemic Chemotherapy

Regimen

Three drug regimen of carboplatin, vincristine and etoposide given in 3–6 cycles

— CHLA doses: carboplatin (13 mg/kg/day), vincristine (0.05 mg/kg/day), etoposide (5.0 mg/kg/day); all 3 drugs given for 2 sequential days
— For patients <6 months of age, carboplatin and etoposide are given at 50% dose (vincristine not given)

Concomitant Focal Therapy

— Begin laser consolidation after 1–2 cycles; retina should be attached
— Wait 2–3 cycles for tumors in the macula to allow for maximal regression

Causes of failure

— Resistant subretinal or vitreous seeding (recurrence rate 46–62%)
— Recurrence of original tumor(s) after completion of chemoreduction
— Development of new retinal tumors

Complications

— Short-term side effects: fatigue, nausea and vomiting, leukopenia, thrombocytopenia, anemia, neutropenic fever
— Ototoxicity in 0–17% of patients with therapeutic doses of carboplatin, highest risk in children <6 months
— Acute myelogenous leukemia (AML) has been identified in 12 patients in a nationwide survey

5. Periocular Chemotherapy Injection

— 50% success with vitreous seeding in early studies, lower success rate with increased clinical usage
— Complications:

    – Rare: optic nerve atrophy
    – Common: ocular motility restriction and orbital fat atrophy

— Not currently used at most centers in the U.S.

6. Selective Intra-Arterial Chemotherapy (IAC)

— First reported by Abramson and Gobin from Memorial Sloan–Kettering Cancer Center (MSKCC) in 2008, modified from an intra-carotid technique used by Kaneko in the 1980's

Indications

— Available as salvage therapy in most modern retinoblastoma centers
— Used as primary therapy for select Group D and E tumors, alone or in combination with systemic chemotherapy at several centers including MSKCC

Technique

Micro-cathether delivers chemotherapy at ostium of ophthalmic artery: 3.0–7.5 mg of melphalan per treatment (infused over 30 min); multidrug regimen of carboplatin, melphalan and topotecan used in salvage cases

— 3–6 infusions per eye 1 month apart administered by an interventional radiologist

Efficacy

— 4 year data from the Abramson group demonstrated a 81.7% rate of avoiding enucleation or radiation when used as primary treatment, 58.4% when used as salvage

Complications

— Minor and transient: periocular edema, eyelash loss, forehead hyperemia
— Rare and serious: retinal and choroidal artery occlusion, vitreous hemorrhage
— Systemic neutropenia has been reported in a minority of children after IAC
— Transfusions are rarely necessary after IAC

7. Intravitreal Chemotherapy (IVC)

Indications

— Isolated vitreous seeding after primary treatment with systemic or intra-arterial chemotherapy (not effective for retinal tumors)
— Success rate in treating vitreous seeding 87–100% in series by Shields and Munier

Protocol

— important safety measures include:

(1) Ultrasound biomicroscopy (UBM) to rule out pars plana involvement
(2) Pre-injection paracentesis
(3) Post-injection cryotherapy at the site of injection
(4) Injection performed with 32 or 33 ga needle away from site of seeding
(5) Post-injection topical vigamox and distilled water advocated by some groups for possible antiproliferative or tumorcidal effects

— Melphalan doses 20–40 mcg every 7 to 30 days
— Risk of ERG changes 30 mcg and above
— Dose of 20 mcg in 0.05 cc used in most cases
— No cases of extraocular spread in the U.S.

Complications

— Common: peripheral pigment changes or chorioretinal atrophy near site of injection
— Rare: vitreous hemorrhage, retinal detachment, ocular phthisis

8. Laser Therapy

Indications

1) Consolidation of large tumors after systemic chemotherapy (i.e. chemoreduction)

  — Continue until all type II regression (fish flesh) has been eradicated

2) Small peripheral or posterior tumors as primary treatment

  — All new tumors receive at least 3 treatment sessions (2–4 week intervals)

3) Small tumor recurrences within or adjacent to scars

  — All recurrent tumors receive 3 treatment sessions (2–4 week intervals)

Wavelength options

— Green argon (532 nm), better absorption when no RPE under tumor
— Red infrared diode (810 nm) deeper penetration vs argon when RPE present

Treatment parameters

— Completely cover the tumor with 1 spot size margin for peripheral tumors, $\frac{1}{2}$ spot size margin with tumors in the macula
— Argon settings: 250–600 mW, durations of 300–500 ms.
— Diode settings: 250–600 mW, 9000 ms duration/50 ms interval (continuous mode)

Efficacy

— For tumor with diameter <3.0 mm and thickness <2.0 mm, control rate 85–95%

Complications

— Burns of the iris at pupillary margin
— Focal lens opacities
— Subhyaloid and vitreous hemorrhage

9. Cryotherapy

Indications:

— Small peripheral tumors <3.0 mm in diameter and <2.0 mm in thickness
— Small tumors with localized vitreous seeding at apex
— Consolidation of larger peripheral tumors in conjunction with or after systemic chemotherapy (i.e. chemoreduction)
— Continue until all type II regression (fish flesh) has been eradicated

Treatment parameters

— Using indirect ophthalmoscopy guidance, depress the cryoprobe tip on the sclera
— Once the probe is directly beneath the tumor, freezing is initiated, and the ice ball maintained until it encompasses the entire tumor mass
— After the treatment covers the apex of the tumor for 1–2 mm, the ice ball is allowed to thaw, and this freeze–thaw cycle repeated for a total of two or three applications
— To avoid iatrogenic injury, do not move the probe on the sclera until the ice ball has completely resolved

Efficacy

— For small peripheral tumors, 70–95% cure rate with cryotherapy
— Recurrences may occur in the cryotherapy scar and present as translucent or white nodules

Complications

— Retinal breaks and rhegmatogenous retinal detachment can result from a combination of the atrophic retina and vitreous traction, particularly at the edges of calcified scars
— Vitreous hemorrhage
— Hypotony from extensive anterior cryotherapy
— Post-treatment transient chemosis and perio-orbital edema for 2 to 3 days is common and expected especially with extensive treatment

10. Brachytherapy

Indications

— Focal tumors too large for cryotherapy or laser treatment
— No increased risk of second cancers or orbital hypoplasia
— The ideal candidate:

  – Focal tumor >2 mm but <6 mm in thickness
  – Any vitreous or subretinal seeds <3 mm from tumor margin
  – Tumor margin >2 disc diameters away from the macula or optic nerve

Treatment parameters

— Iodine-125 used in the United States: 4,000 to 4,500 cGy to the apex of the tumor at a rate of 50–150 cGy/hour
— Ruthenium-106 used in Europe

Efficacy

— Primary therapy: tumor control rate 80–95%
— Salvage therapy: 50–60% tumor control rate

Complications

— Radiation retinopathy 27%, papillopathy 26%, cataract 31%, intraocular hemorrhage 29% and neovascular glaucoma in 11%

11. External Beam Radiotherapy (EBR)

— EBR can treat tumors in the posterior pole without worsening central vision
— Useful modality to treat both eyes simultaneously

Indications

— Used mainly as salvage therapy in children >18 months of age (younger children at risk for second cancers and orbital hypoplasia)
— Avoid using EBR in eyes with dismal visual potential
— Avoid EBR if there is good visual potential in the contralateral eye

Treatment parameters

— CHLA protocol: total dose of 36 Gy of Intensity modulated radiotherapy (IMRT), increasing the dose up to 42 Gy if there is a large tumor load
— 180 to 200 cGy daily fractions, five times per week
— General anesthesia required for each session

Efficacy

— Primary therapy, tumor control rates of 50–95% (depending on RE stage). The globe preservation rate is 95% for group I–II eyes treated with EBR, but only about 50% for eyes in groups IV and V

  – Salvage rate after chemoreduction 70–80%.

Complications

— Second cancer risk in patients with hereditary retinoblastoma treated with external beam radiation from 1914–1984 approximately 50%
— Non-ocular cancers observed in survivors of germinal retinoblastoma include, in order of most common to least common: soft tissue sarcomas, ostegenic sarcomas of the skull and long bones, pineoblastomas, cutaneous melanomas, brain tumors, Hodgkin's disease, lung cancer, breast cancer, and skin cancer
— Orbital and midfacial hypoplasia
— Optic neuropathy, retinal vascular occlusion, vitreous hemorrhage and neovascular glaucoma
— Intensity-modulated Radiation Therapy (IMRT) is a more focused treatment and may lessen bony hypoplasia
— Common findings after EBR include keratitis sicca, cataract 85% of eyes over 12–49 months of follow-up, loss of lashes, transient skin erythema
— Severe keratitis sicca is very common in the first 3 months after treatment and we recommend performing prophylactic silicone punctual plug placement in all children undergoing EBR to reduce photophobia and ocular discomfort

12. Proton or Particle Beam Irradiation

— Limited availability and limited published data
— Offered in limited centers
— May offer more localized delivery of radiation than other modes of external beam radiation with sparing of radiation to the normal bony structures of the orbit and anterior segment of the eye
— Local failure reported in eyes with diffuse seeding

13. Enucleation

— Most common treatment for retinoblastoma worldwide, curative in 96–98% cases
— MRI should always be done preoperatively to rule out >5 mm of optic nerve enhancement which would require neo-adjuvant chemotherapy
— These high risk histologic features of enucleated eye would require systemic chemotherapy to minimize risk of extraocular tumor recurrence and/or metastasis

   1. Choroidal invasion of tumor
   2. Invasion of tumor into the optic nerve beyond the lamina cribosa

Indications

— Unilateral Group D disease
— Any Group E eye
— Active tumor following the completion of primary therapy in a blind eye
— Active tumor with obscured media (vitreous hemorrhage, cataract)

Surgical technique

— Avoid perforations of the globe
— Obtain a long section of optic nerve of at least 12–15 mm.
— Acceptable implants: silicone, hydroxyapatite, Medpor and dermis fat graft
— Silicone spheres:

   – Widely available, rare complications, acceptable motility

— Porous implants (hydroxyapatite and Medpor):

   – Low rates of implant migration but higher rates of exposure
   – Potential for better motility if the implant is pegged

— <6 months (16–18 mm), 6–24 months (18 mm), >24 months (19–20 mm)
— After 4–6 weeks, patients fitted with a prosthesis by ocularist
— Monitor closely for 12 months for orbital recurrence or systemic disease

14. Treatment Overview

Enucleation

— Unilateral Group D
— Any Group E eye (unilateral or bilateral)

Chemoreduction or systemic chemotherapy

— Unilateral or bilateral Groups B to D
— High risk features of unilateral Groups D or E enucleated eye

Focal treatment (laser/cryotherapy)

— Primary treatment: Group A
— Combined treatment: during chemoreduction: Groups B to D
— Salvage treatment: small retinal tumor recurrences: Groups B to D

Brachytherapy

— Primary treatment: unilateral Groups B or C (peripheral)
— Salvage treatment: large tumor recurrences without seeding (peripheral or posterior)

Intra-arterial chemotherapy infusion (IAC)

— Primary therapy: unilateral Group D
— Salvage therapy: unilateral retinal recurrence or combined retinal and Vitreous recurrence after systemic chemotherapy
— Limited to patient >6 months of age due to vascular access

External Beam radiation (EBR)

— Salvage only after chemoreduction or IAC failure
— >18 months of age
— Bilateral retinal or combined retinal and vitreous recurrences
— Unilateral retinal or combined retinal and vitreous recurrence if better seeing eye

Intravitreal chemotherapy injections (IVC)

— First choice for salvage of isolated vitreous seeding after chemoreduction or EBR
— Unilateral or bilateral, no age limit
— Not effective for retinal tumor recurrences

15. Genetic Testing

— Mutation can be identified to 85% of familial cases
— May be useful to screen family members who may be at risk
— May be useful to identify germline mutation in isolated cases of unilateral retinoblastoma

16. Post-treatment Surveillance

— Exam under anesthesia is performed till age 6 to rule out new local tumor recurrence
— MRI scan of head and orbit every 6 to 12 months is performed for tumors with history of optic nerve involvement and bilateral cases to rule out CNS tumors (e.g. pinealomas)

References

1. Kim JW, Abramson DH, Dunkel IJ. Current management strategies for intraocular retinoblastoma. *Drugs* 2007;67(15):2173–2185.
2. Berry JL, Jubran R, Kim JW, *et al.* Long-term outcomes of Group D eyes in bilateral retinoblastoma patients treated with chemoreduction and low-dose IMRT salvage. *Pediatr Blood Cancer* 2013;60(4):688–693.
3. Murphree AL, Villablanca JG, Deegan 3rd, WF, *et al.* Chemotherapy plus local treatment in the management of intraocular retinoblastoma. *Arch Ophthalmol* 1996;114(11):1348–1356.
4. Wilson MW, Rodriguez-Galindo C, Haik BG, *et al.* Multiagent chemotherapy as neoadjuvant treatment for multifocal intraocular retinoblastoma. *Ophthalmol* 2001;108(11):2106–2114; discussion 14–15.
5. Abramson DH, Dunkel IJ, Brodie SE, *et al.* A phase I/II study of direct intraarterial (ophthalmic artery) chemotherapy with melphalan for intraocular retinoblastoma initial results. *Ophthalmol* 2008;115(8):1398–404, 404 e1.
8. Gobin YP, Dunkel IJ, Marr BP, *et al.* Intra-arterial chemotherapy for the management of retinoblastoma: four-year experience. *Arch Ophthalmol* 2011;129(6):732–737.
9. Munier FL, Soliman S, Moulin AP, *et al.* Profiling safety of intravitreal injections for retinoblastoma using an anti-reflux procedure and sterilisation of the needle track. *Br J Ophthalmol* 2012;96(8):1084–1087.
10. Abramson DH, Schefler AC. Transpupillary thermotherapy as initial treatment for small intraocular retinoblastoma: technique and predictors of success. *Ophthalmol* 2004;111(5):984–991.
11. Abramson DH, Ellsworth RM, Rozakis GW. Cryotherapy for retinoblastoma. *Arch Ophthalmol* 1982;100(8):1253–1256.
12. Schueler AO, Fluhs D, Anastassiou G, *et al.* Beta-ray brachytherapy with 106 Ru plaques for retinoblastoma. *Int J Radiat Oncol Biol Phys* 2006;65(4):1212–1221.
13. Merchant TE, Gould CJ, Wilson MW, *et al.* Episcleral plaque brachytherapy for retinoblastoma. *Pediatr Blood Cancer* 2004;43(2):134–139.
14. Wong FL, Boice Jr., JD, Abramson DH, *et al.* Cancer incidence after retinoblastoma. Radiation dose and sarcoma risk. *JAMA* 1997;278(15):1262–1267.
15. Abramson DH, Frank CM. Second nonocular tumors in survivors of bilateral retinoblastoma: a possible age effect on radiation-related risk. *Ophthalmol* 1998;105(4):573–579; discussion 9–80.
16. Abramson DH, Jereb B, Ellsworth RM. External beam radiation for retinoblastoma. *Bull N Y Acad Med* 1981;57(9):787–803.
17. Abramson DH, Ellsworth RM. The surgical management of retinoblastoma. *Ophthalmic Surg* 1980;11(9):596–598.
18. Kim JW, Kathpalia V, Dunkel IJ, *et al.* Orbital recurrence of retinoblastoma following enucleation. *Br J Ophthalmol* 2009;93(4):463–467.

Chapter 26: Choroidal Nevus and Melanocytoma

Susanna S. Park

CHOROIDAL NEVUS

1. Incidence

5% of Caucasian Population (range 2 to 6%)
1% non-Caucasians (range 0.4 to 1.4%)

2. Clinical Features

Usually asymptomatic

Size: <6.0 mm basal diameter (distinct or ill-defined border)
Ultrasound: flat to <2 mm thickness (medium to high reflectivity)
Pigmentation: grey-brown to amelanotic
Fundus appearance: hypo pigmented ring at base; overlying drusen (50%)
Growth: possible during puberty and young adulthood

— progressive rapid growth suggests malignant transformation

3. Differential Diagnosis & Clinical features

a. Melanoma: >2 mm thickness, low internal reflectivity, growth
b. Metastasis: amelanotic, rapid growth, high internal reflectivity
c. Hemangioma: orange pigmentation, high internal reflectivity
d. Osteoma: calcificationdetected by ultrasound or CT scan
e. Hypertrophy of the retinal pigment epithelium: flat, black to dark-brown

f. Chorioretinal atrophy or scar: atrophy of overlying RPE and retina by OCT

g. Sub retinal or sub-RPE hemorrhage: decrease with observation

4. Initial Evaluation

a. History

    i.   Determine if new change

       1. Compare with any prior fundus photographs available

       2. Any associated new visual symptoms

          — new change in visual acuity, metamorphopsia, flashes/floaters

b. Eye Examination: document Appearance of Nevus

    i.   Note Location in Fundus

       1. Distance from Disc & Fovea

    ii. Note basal diameter (Widest dimension × 90° to widest dimension).

    iii. Pigmentation

          — orange, amelanotic, overlying drusen, etc.

    iv. Elevation versus flat

    v. Any associated sub retinal fluid or hemorrhage

c. Diagnostic Test: baseline and serial follow-up for comparison (Figure 1).

    i.   Color Fundus Photography

    ii. Ultrasonography

       1. B-scan: measurement accuracy may be limited for minimally elevated lesion

       2. A-scan: rule out following risk factors for malignant transformation

          a. Tumor thickness: >2 mm

          b. Low Internal reflectivity

    iii. Spectral-domain OCT

       1. Feature at risk factor for malignant transformation:

          a. Presence of sub retinal fluid

       2. Chronic benign findings

          a. Overlying retinal cystoid changes

          b. Overlying RPE atrophy

iv. Enhanced Depth Imaging SD-OCT (Spectralis)

1. More accurate measure of tumor thickness than Ultrasound.

   — Usually lower thickness than A-scan

2. Thinning of overly choriocapillaris: common feature

v. Fluorescein Angiogram

1. Usually not needed: variable finding
2. Useful to rule out simulating lesions or associated Choroidal Neovascular membrane (CNVM)

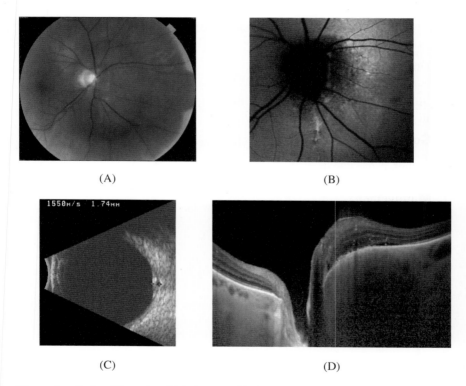

(A)   (B)

(C)   (D)

Figure 1.   Peripapillary choroidal pigmented lesion with high risk features for malignant transformation. (A) Fundus photograph showing the lesion wrapped around the optic disc with some orange pigmentation. (B) Autofluoresence showed diffuse marked hyperfluorescence. (C) B-scan ultrasonography shows the lesion is elevated with thickness of 1.7 mm. (D) Spectral-domain optical coherence tomography showing the choroidal involvement around the optic nerve and trace amount of sub retinal fluid that is forming over the lesion.

vi. Autofluoresence

1. Detect orange pigmentation as bright hyperfluorescence

5. Risk of Malignant Transformation

Incidence: caucasians: 1/8,800 per year

A. Risk factors for Malignant Transformation: rule of five

    i. Orange Pigmentation
    ii. Sub retinal Fluid
    iii. Visual Symptoms
    iv. Elevation >2 mm
    v. Near Disc Margin (<3 mm)

B. Other poor prognostic signs

    i. Low Internal reflectivity on ultrasonography
    ii. Rapid Growth

6. Good Prognostic Clinical Features

Flat tumor, chronic features-overlying drusen.

7. Management and Follow-up of Nevus

a. Benign Low Risk Nevus

Annual follow-up examination and imaging as needed.

b. Nevus "At Risk"

    i. Consider Referral to Specialist or
    ii. Close Follow-up 3 to 6 months for >1.5 years, then 6 to 12 months.

    — Slow growth of nevus is not necessarily sign of malignant transformation (30% slight growth over 7 to15 years).
    — Signs of Malignant Transformation.

        i. Rapid Growth of lesion
        ii. Rule of Five

c. Intermediate Lesion/Small Melanoma (Lesions with 2 to 3 mm thickness).

    — can be observed every 3 months for signs of progressive growth and change especially if close to disc and macula before considering treatment.

— COMS Study: mortality rate of small melanomas was 6% at 5 years and 15% at 8 years overall (but only 20% of the deaths were from metastasis).

8. Management of Non-malignant Complications

— Incidence: rare
— Examples:

Choroidal neovascularization
Pigment epithelial detachment
Sub macular fluid

— Diagnostic testing: Fluorescein angiography and OCT.
— Treatment options:

Intravitreal avastin
Photodynamic therapy
Laser therapy
Radiation if worrisome for malignant transformation.

MELANOCYTOMA

1. Incidence

0.5%

2. Clinical Features

Locations: Optic disc >>> choroid > ciliary body > iris > retina
Association: 50 to 85% with choroidal component, 30% retinal component

8% Ocular melanocytosis
7% Racial melanocytosis

Pigmentation: usually dark brown to black but rarely less pigmented
Appearance: feathery border from retinal nerve fiber layer involvement
Size: average 2 mm diameter × 1 mm thickness
Unilateral (99%)
Ethnicity: all
Female > Male
Age of diagnosis: mean 50 years
Asymptomatic (75%) but enlarged blind spot (90%).
Afferent papillary defect (9%)

Fluorescein or ICG Angiography:

Blocked hypofluorescence of lesion from melanin (Figure 2)
Intrinsic tumor vascularity might suggest risk of malignant transformation

OCT: hyperreflective anterior tumor surface with marked shadowing (Figure 2(c))

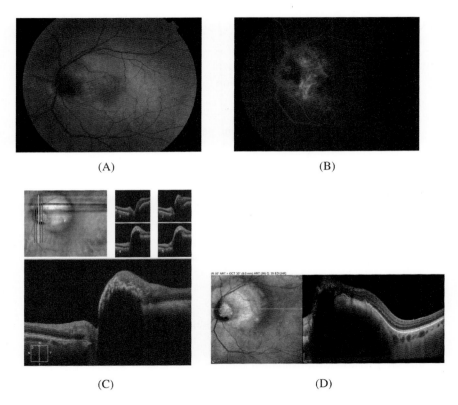

(A) (B)

(C) (D)

Figure 2. Melanocytoma with associated elevated choroidal component. (A) Red-free photography showing the melanocytoma of the optic disc with adjacent choroidal lesion involving the macula. (B) Fluorescein angiogram showing hypofluorescence of the melanocytoma of the optic disc with marked hyperfluorescence of the adjacent peripapillary lesion. (C) OCT of the disc showing the hyperreflective superficial layer with deeper marked shadowing associated with the melanocytoma. (D) EDI-OCT of the peripapillary choroidal lesion showing marked elevation with trace overlying subretinal fluid suspicious for malignant transformation to melanoma.

2. Clinical Course

a. Stable size usually; may increase pigmentation over time
b. Slight benign growth (11% over 5 years, 32% over 10 years)
c. Disc edema (25%) with usually good visual acuity
d. Retinal exudation or fluid (12%): main reason for vision loss
e. Retinal hemorrhage (5%)
f. Central retinal artery or vein occlusion (2 to 4%)
g. Vitreous seeding (4 to 5%)
    Choroidal neovascularization: rare
h. Malignant transformation (1 to 2%)

    i.   Risk factors: choroidal component, vitreous seeding, rapid progressive growth, thickness >1.5 mm, vision loss

i. Spontaneous necrosis: rare

    i.   May lead to severe vision loss and pain

3. Differential Diagnosis

a. Malignant Uveal Melanoma
b. Hyperplasia of the RPE
c. Adenoma of the RPE
d. Metastatic Melanoma of the Optic Disc

4. Management

a. Baseline Imaging: documentation of diagnosis

    i.   Fundus photography
    ii. OCT to check for exudation and tumor elevation
    iii. Perimetry to evaluate for blind spots

b. Annual follow-up examination or sooner as needed

    i.   Repeat photography, OCT and perimetry, as needed

References

1. Singh AD, Kalyani P, Topham A. Estimating the risk of malignant transformation of a choroidal nevus. *Ophthalmol* 2005;112:1784–1789.
2. Shields CL, Furuta M, Berman EL, *et al*. Choroidal nevus transformation into melanoma: Analysis of 2514 consecutive cases. *Arch Ophthalmol* 2009;127:981–987.
3. Mashayekhi A, Siu S, Shields CL, *et al*. Slow enlargement of choroidal nevi: A long-term follow-up study. *Ophthalmol* 2011;118:382–388.
4. Shields CL, Cater J, Shields JA, *et al*. Combination of clinical factors predictive of growth of small choroidal melanocytic tumors. *Arch Ophthalmol* 2000;118:360–364.
5. Collaborative Ocular Melanoma Study (COMS) Group. Factors predictive of growth and treatment of small choroidal melanoma. COMS report No 5. *Arch Ophthalmol* 1997;115:1537–1544.
6. Shields CL, Kaliki S, Rojanaporn D, *et al*. Enhanced depth imaging optical coherence tomography of small choroidal melanoma: Comparison with choroidal nevus. *Arch Ophthalmol* 2012;130:850–856.
7. Lee CS, Bae JH, Jeon IH, *et al*. Melanocytoma of the optic disk in the Korean population. *Retina* 2010;30:1714–1720.
8. Shields JA, Demirci H, Mashayekhi A, *et al*.Melanocytoma of optic disc in 115 cases: The 2004 Samuel Johnson Memoral Lecture, part 1. *Ophthalmology* 2004;111:1739–1746.
9. Shields JA, Demirci H, Mashayekhi A, *et al*. Melanocytoma of the optic disk: A review.*Surv Ophthalmol* 2006;51:93–104.
10. Shields CL, Perez B, Benavides R, *et al*. Optical coherence tomography of the optic disc melanocytoma in 15 cases. *Retina* 2008;28:441–446.

Chapter 27: Choroidal Melanoma

Susanna S. Park

1. Incidence

a. Most common primary intraocular malignancy

   i. Choroidal tumors account for 80% of uveal melanomas

b. 5 to 7 new cases per million per year

   i. much rarer than skin melanoma

   ii. accounts for 12% of all melanoma cases

c. Risk of malignant transformation of choroidal nevus: 1 in 8,800 per year

2. Risk Factors for Ocular Melanoma

a. Older age (Middle-age)

b. Caucasian (Fair skin and light-colored eyes)

c. History of sun exposure

d. Ocular melanocytosis (Ocular melanoma risk: 1%)

3. Clinical Features

a. Presenting Symptoms: 33% asymptomatic

   i. New change in vision or metamorphopsia

   ii. New flashes or floaters

   iii. Chronic "red eye": sentinel vessels (Figure 1)

b. Pigmentation: variable, 25% amelanotic

c. Shape of tumor elevation

    i. Dome-shaped: most common

    ii. Mushroom-shaped: seen after tumor breaks through Bruch's membrane into sub retinal space

    iii. Diffuse: <5 mm choroidal elevation and >25% of choroidal involvement

        1. May simulate large choroidal nevus

        2. Increased risk of extra scleral extension

d. Associated ocular findings

    i. Exudative retinal detachment

    ii. Extra scleral tumor extension

    iii. Sentinel vessels: if ciliary body involvement of tumor (Figure 1)

    iv. Lens opacification or subluxation for anterior tumor

    v. Glaucoma

        1. Iris neovascularization or

        2. Tumor invasion of angle

    vi. Vitreous hemorrhage: usually associated with tumor invasion into retina

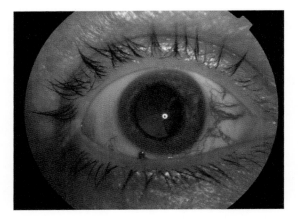

Figure 1. Slit lamp photograph of an eye with a large nasal ciliochoroidal melanoma visible through the pupil. Prominent sentinel vessels are noted under the nasal conjunctiva.

4. Diagnostic Testing

a. Ultrasonography: >99% diagnostic accuracy (Figure 2)

    i. A-scan: medium to low internal reflectivity

   ii. B-scan: choroidal mass with acoustic hollowness

       1. Possible associated retinal detachment

       2. Possible associated extra scleral extension

b. Fluorescein angiography

    i. Mottled hyperfluorescence with late staining of mass

   ii. Not diagnostic finding except "double-circulation" of tumor

       1. Seen in amelanotic mushroom-shaped tumor from concurrent retinal and choroidal tumor circulation

       2. May be seen more prominently using ICG

c. Fundus Autofluoresence (AF): variable

       1. Increased AF: small or amelanotic melanomas

       2. Decreased AF: large melanoma

d. Orbital CT or MRI scan

    i. To delineate extent of extra scleral or orbital involvement

   ii. Useful for large tumors with suspected gross extra scleral tumor extension

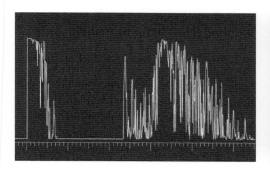 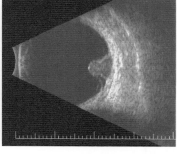

(A)   (B)

Figure 2. Ultrasound of an eye with a choroidal melanoma showing (A) the low internal reflectivity of the tumor on A-scan and (B) a mushroom-shaped mass with acoustic hollowness and associated retinal detachment on B-scan.

e. Fine needle tumor biopsy

   i. Transcleral or transvitreal using 25 to 27-gauge needle
  ii. Not needed for diagnosis except for atypical cases
 iii. Useful for genetic or chromosomal analysis for prognosis.

    1. Genetic profile of tumor (Castle Bioscience)

      a. Class I: <5% risk of metastasis over 5 years
      b. Class II: 80 to 90% risk of metastasis over 5 years
      c. BAP1 Mutation: subclass of Class II

        i. Increased metastasis risk
       ii. May increase risk of other cancers if germline mutation

    2. Chromosomal analysis of tumor (Impact Genetics)

      a. Poor prognosis changes

        i. Chromosome 3 loss
       ii. Chromosome 8q gain
      iii. Chromosome 1p loss

      b. Good prognosis changes

        i. Chromosome 6p gain

5. Metastasis Screening: At Baseline and Every 6 to 12 Months

a. LIVER: most common site of metastasis (60 to 94%)

   i. Review of systems: nausea, abdominal pain, weight loss
  ii. Liver screening with liver function test, MRI, or abdominal ultrasound.

    1. Unable to detect lesions <1 mm in size (micro metastasis)

b. LUNG: second most common site of metastasis (46 to 7%)

   i. Chest X-ray
  ii. CT scan if abnormal Chest X-ray

c. BONE: 29 to 7% site of metastasis
d. SKIN: <24% site of metastasis
e. CNS: 2% site of metastasis

6. Management of Ocular Melanoma

a. Particle Beam Irradiation: >95% local tumor control

   i. Homogeneous delivery of radiation within tumor
   ii. Can treat large tumors
   iii. Minimal lateral spread of radiation
   iv. Availability limited to few clinical centers

b. Brachytherapy: up to 90% local tumor control (COMS study)

   i. More universally available
   ii. Ideal for tumors <9 mm thickness, <18 mm diameter
   iii. Radiation dose highest at point of contact with plaque

c. Enucleation

   i. Reserved for eyes with limited visual potential, very large tumors, diffuse tumors or for patients with poor expected follow-up
   ii. COMS study showed no survival benefit over brachytherapy for medium tumors

d. Surgical Tumor Resection: reserved for select cases

   i. Endoresection with pars planar vitrectomy is reserved for posterior pole tumors where visual preservation is priority

      1. Limited long-term follow-up data available
      2. Residual intraocular tumor cells noted in enucleated eyes

   ii. Partial Lamellar Sclerouvectomy

      1. For localized peripheral tumors >6 mm height
      2. Risk of suprachoroidal hemorrhage and retinal detachment

   iii. Exenteration: for orbital extension of tumor

e. Laser Treatment: reserved for small growing posterior pole tumors but limited follow-up data, reported lower success rate than radiation for tumor control

   i. Argon laser photocoagulation
   ii. Trans pupillary thermotherapy
   iii. Photodynamic therapy: amelanotic tumors

f. Observation with close follow-up (see Chapter 26 on Choroidal nevus)

   i. Small melanomas <2 mm in height with overlying drusen and lack of sub retinal fluid or orange pigmentation

ii. Metastatic ocular melanoma

1. Refer to medical oncology to discuss systemic therapy

7. Long-term Follow-up

a. Ocular evaluation every 6 to 12 months indefinitely to evaluate for local tumor control
b. Metastatic screening every 6 to 12 months indefinitely

   i. No standardized screening protocol

      1. Liver screening: blood test, ultrasound, or MRI
      2. Lung screening: chest X-ray

   ii. May refer to medical oncology for high risk patients

8. Prognosis

a. Risk of metastasis increases with duration of follow-up (Table 1)
b. Other risk factors associated with increased risk of metastasis

   i. Larger tumor size at diagnosis
   ii. Age of patient
   iii. Males
   iv. Ciliary body involvement
   v. Epithelioid cell tumor
   vi. High risk Genetic/Chromosomal alterations in tumor

Table 1. Long-term prognosis of treated ocular melanoma based on tumor size at the time of diagnosis (Shields, *arch ophthalmol* 2009).

Tumor Type	Tumor Thickness, Basal Diameter (mm)	5 Year Mortality (%)	20 Year Mortality (%)
Small	1–3 mm, <5 mm	6	20
Medium	3–8 mm, 5–16 mm	14	37
Large	>8 mm, >16 mm	35	67

9. Metastatic Disease: Prognosis and Treatment

i. No proven therapy
ii. Poor prognosis (mean survival 6 to 12 months)
iii. Local chemotherapy and surgical resection being explored
iv. Adjuvant chemotherapy and liver radiation being explored for high risk patients but no proven efficacy

References

1. Collaborative Ocular Melanoma Study Group. Accuracy of diagnosis of choroidal melanomas in the Collaborative Ocular Melanoma Study. COMS Report No. 1. *Arch Ophthalmol* 1990;108:1268–1273.

2. Collaborative Ocular Melanoma Study Group. Assessment of metastatic disease status at death in 435 patients with large choroidal melanoma in the Collaborative Ocular Melanoma Study. COMS Report No. 15. *Arch Ophthalmol* 2001;119:670–676.

3. Collaborative Ocular Melanoma Study Group. The COMS randomized trial of Iodine 125 brachytherapy for choroidal melanoma, III: Initial mortality findings. COMS Report No. 18. *Arch Ophthalmol* 2001;119:969–982.

4. Damato BE, *et al.* Translating uveal melanoma cytogenetics into clinical care. *Arch Ophthalmol* 2009;127:423–429.

5. Gragoudas ES, Egan KM, Seddon JM, *et al.* Intraocular recurrences of uveal melanoma after proton beam irradiation. *Ophthalmol* 1992;99:760–766.

6. Habour JW, Onken MD, Roberson EDO, *et al.* Frequent mutation of BAP1 in metastasizing uveal melanomas. *Science* 2010;330:1410–1413.

7. Shields JA, Shields CL, Ehya H, *et al.* Fine needle aspiration biopsy of suspected intraocular tumors. The 1992 Urwick Lecture. *Ophthalmol* 1993;100:1677–1684.

8. Shields CL, Minoru F, Archana T, *et al.* Metastasis of uveal melanoma millimeter-by-millimeter in 8033 cosecutive eyes. *Arch Ophthalmol* 2009;127:989–998.

9. The COMS randomized trial of iodine 125 brachytherapy for choroidal meleanoma: IV. Local treatment failure and enucleation in the first 5 years after brachytherapy. COMS report no. 19. *Ophthalmol* 2002;109:2197–2206.

Chapter 28: Choroidal Metastasis

Susanna S. Park

1. Choroidal Metastasis

- Metastasis is the most common intraocular malignancy
- Choroid is the most common uveal location for intraocular metastasis (90%) due to the high vascular supply

  - Iris (9%) and ciliary body (2%) involvement can also occur but less common

- Most common primary site of malignancy with choroidal metastatic involvement

  - Women: breast carcinoma (68%)
  - Men: lung carcinoma (40%)
  - Other common primary cancers with choroidal metastasis

    - Prostate, kidney, thyroid, GI tract cancers

2. Clinical Signs and Symptoms

- Usually present with painless subacute vision loss or new flashes or floaters

  - Asymptomatic (11%)
  - Typically unilateral but can be bilateral,
  - There may be significant associated eye pain (7%)

    - May not be explained on clinical examination
    - Likely due to perineural invasion of tumor

  - Eye finding may present signs of systemic malignancy in some patients (25%)
  - May be a sign of occult systemic malignancy where the primary site is never identified (10 to 18%)

Fundus findings

- Amelanotic choroidal mass with possible associated pigment changes
- Posterior pole location typically (90%)
- May by multifocal or bilateral
- Relatively fast growing
- Associated serous retinal detachment (64%)

  o May become bullous especially in more advanced cases (Figure 1)

3. Diagnostic Testing

- Ultrasonography

  o Choroidal mass with high internal reflectivity supports diagnosis but findings are not specific to metastatic tumors
  o Associated serous retinal detachment may be seen
  o Tumor dimensions are recorded as a parameter to follow

- Fluorescein angiogram, Indocyanine Green(ICG) and Fundus photography

  o Useful to rule out other causes of serous retinal detachment or choroidal thickening and to document extent of pathology

- Optical Coherence Tomography (OCT)

  o Useful to detect associated sub retinal fluid
  o EDI mode will improve visualization of the choroidal mass (Figure 1D)

- Whole body Positron Emission Tomography-Computerized Tomography (PET-CT) Scan

  o To determine extent of metastatic disease and/or identify site of primary malignancy
  o Typically ordered in conjunction with medical oncologist

- Mammogram or Chest X-ray

  o Useful screening, if no known history of systemic malignancy

- Tumor biopsy

  o Usually not necessary unless the primary tumor cannot be identified
  o Can be performed as a fine needle biopsy or partial tumor resection
  o Biopsy diagnostic sensitivity of 100% and specificity of 98%

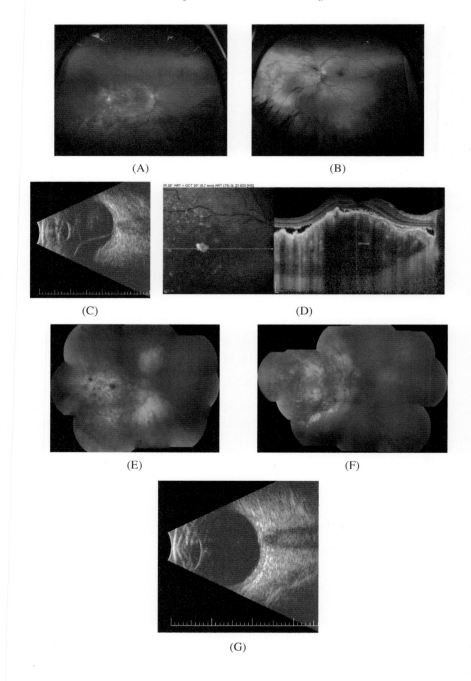

(A)   (B)

(C)   (D)

(E)   (F)

(G)

←

Figure 1. (*Figure on facing page*)   Choroidal metastasis both eyes from metastatic breast carcinoma. Fundus photographs at presentation using the Optos wide-angle camera showing a large macular lesion with associated bullous inferior serous retinal detachment in the right eye (A) and **a** large nasal lesion in the left eye (B). B-scan ultrasonography at presentation shows a diffuse infiltrating choroidal mass with associated retinal detachment (C). Enhanced depth imaging mode of macula OCT of the right eye shows the choroidal mass which can be measured (D). Associated subretinal fluid involving the macula is appreciated. Following systemic chemotherapy, the choroidal lesions in both eyes completely regressed. Fundus photograph montage shows the residual pigment changes in the area of the regressed choroidal tumors in the right (E) and left (F) eyes. B-scan ultrasonography of the right eye following treatment shows complete resolution of the retinal detachment with no measurable mass (G).

4. Treatment

- Systemic chemotherapy is the primary treatment since choroidal involvement is a sign of systemic metastatic disease
- Local radiotherapy may be used in conjunction, in cases of resistance to systemic chemotherapy

  o External beam radiation may be performed in bilateral cases or in cases with concurrent brain metastasis
  o Proton beam or plaque therapy may be considered in cases of solitary unilateral choroidal mass

- Enucleation can be considered in unilateral advanced cases with limited visual potential especially if associated with intractable eye pain

5. Management and Follow-up

- Close follow-up every 1 to 2 months during administration of systemic chemotherapy is important to monitor for treatment response or lack of response

  o Serial fundus photography, OCT and ultrasonography are typically performed with comprehensive eye examination
  o Resolution of sub retinal fluid and decrease in tumor height are signs of treatment response
  o New metastatic lesions may be seen which would denote resistant or recurrent disease
  o Serial PET-CT scan is typically ordered by medical oncology

- A team approach is critical with close communication, with, treating medical oncologist and/or radiation oncologist

6. Prognosis

- Various with prognosis of primary malignancy
- Breast cancer with choroidal metastasis is the most common
  - o Prognosis better than other metastatic malignancies:
    - ■ 65% survival at 1 year
    - ■ 25% survival at 5 years

References

1. Shields CL, Shields JA, Gross N, *et al.* Survey of 520 eyes with uveal metastases. *Ophthalmol* 1997;104:1265–1276.
2. Demirci H, Shields CL, Chao A-N, *et al.* Uveal Metastasis from Breast Cancer in 264 Patients. *Am J Ophthalmol* 2003;136(2):264–271.
3. Shields JA, Shields CL, Ehya H, *et al.* Fine needle aspiration biopsy of suspected intraocular tumors. The 1992 Urwick Lecture. *Ophthalmol* 1993;100:1677–1684.
4. BCSC Section 4: Ophthalmic Pathology and Intraocular Tumors. Chapter 20. 2010–2011.
5. Krause L, Bechrakis NE, Kreusel KM, *et al.* Indocyanine green angiography in choroid metastases. *Ophthalmol* 2002; 99(8):617–619.
6. Sobottka B, Schlote T, Krumpaszky HG, *et al.* Choroidal metastases and choroidal melanomas: Comparison of ultrasonographic findings. *Br J Ophthalmol* 1998; 82(2):159–161.

Appendix: Intravitreal Injections

Susanna S. Park

1. Technique

a. Local anesthetic

    i. Proparacaine, tetracaine or 4% lidocaine

    ii. Lidocaine gel

        1. Direct application and/or pluget

    iii. Subconjunctival Lidocaine 2%

        1. Risk scarring of conjunctiva with repeat

b. Digital massage to soften eye if injection volume >0.05 cc

    i. Paracentesis may be needed if volume >0.1 cc

c. 5% Betadine is instilled in the fornix and at site of injection

d. Sterile lid speculum

e. Inject pars planar (3.5–4 mm behind limbus) with 27–32 gauge needle

f. Check visual acuity of at least counting finger

g. Check optic nerve perfusion with indirect ophthalmoscopy

h. Rinse eye with balanced saline solution

i. Apply antibiotic drop or ointment

2. Indications for Intravitreal Injections

a. ENDOPHTHALMITIS TREATMENT

    i. Gram-positive: vancomycin 1 mg/0.1 mL or Clindamycin 500 mcg/0.1 mL, and

    ii. Gram-negative: ceftazidime 2.25 mg/0.1 mL or Amikacin 400 mcg/0.1 mL

    iii. Optional

        1. Anti-fungal: amphotericin 5 to 10 μg/0.1ml, or

        2. Anti-inflammatory: dexamethasone 0.4 mg/0.1ml

b. PNEUMATIC RETINOPEXY: IDEAL VOLUME OF EXPANSILE GAS TO BE INJECTED

    i. 0.3 cc of undiluted gas, or

    ii. 0.05 cc + Volume of aspirated intraocular fluid

c. PNEUMATIC DISPLACEMENT OF SUBMACULAR HEMORRHAGE

    i. tPA: 20 to 50 μg and

    ii. Expansile gas: 0.3 to 0.4 cc undiluted

d. UVEITIS MANAGEMENT

    i. Intravitreal triamcinolone (40 mg/ml)

        1. 1mg to 4 mg in 0.025 to 0.1 cc

            a. Lasts average 3 months

            b. 20 to 25% risk of intraocular pressure elevation

            c. 5% risk of pseudoendophthalmitis with Kenalog

            d. Triescence is preservative-free and FDA-approved for ocular use

    ii. Ozurdex (700 μg dexamethasone injectable slow-release implant)

        1. FDA approved for uveitis treatment

        2. Lasts up to 3 to 6 months

        3. 10 to 15% risk of intraocular pressure elevation

        4. Contraindicated in eyes without an intact posterior lens capsule

    iii. Intravitreal Methotrexate (400 μg in 0.1 cc)

        1. Have been used to treat refractory uveitis with CME

iv. Intravitreal infliximab (Remicade 0.5–1 mg/0.05 cc)

    1. Have been used to treat severe refractory sight-threatening uveitis (Behcets)

    2. Adverse effects noted in nonuveitis eyes: ERG changes, uveitis

e. <u>CYSTOID MACULAR EDEMA (CME) DUE TO RETINAL VEIN OCCLUSION</u>

    i. Intravitreal corticosteroid

        1. Triamcinolone (40 mg/ml)
            a. SCORE Study: 1 mg as effective as 4mg with less glaucoma

        2. Ozurdex: FDA approved for CRVO and BRVO

            a. GENEVA Study: superior to observation or grid laser

    ii. Intravitreal anti-VEGF (Table 1)

        1. Bevacizumab (Avastin, 1.25 mg in 0.05 cc)

            a. Used off-label
            b. Inexpensive

        2. Ranibizumab (Lucentis, 0.5 mg in 0.05 cc)

            a. FDA-approved for CME from CRVO or BRVO
            b. CRUISE and BRAVO Studies: superior to observation or grid laser

        3. Aflibercept (Eylea, 2 mg in 0.05 cc)

            a. FDA-approved for CME from CRVO
            b. GALILEO, COPERNICUS Studies: superior to observation

f. <u>DIABETIC MACULAR EDEMA WITH CENTRAL INVOLVEMENT</u>

    i. Intravitreal anti-VEGF

        1. Bevacizumab (Avastin, 1.25 mg in 0.05 cc): off-label
        2. Ranibuzimab (Lucentis, 0.3 mg in 0.03 cc): FDA-approved lower dose
        3. Aflibercept (Eylea, 2 mg in 0.05 cc)

    ii. Intravitreal corticosteroid

       1. Triamcinolone 1 mg in 0.025 cc
       2. Ozurdex

          a. pseudophakic eyes without glaucoma
          b. eyes with pre-exisiting cataract

g. <u>EXUDATIVE AGE-RELATED MACULAR DEGENERATION</u>

    i. Intravitreal anti-Vascular endothelial growth factor (VEGF)

       1. Bevacizumab (Avastin, 1.25 mg in 0.05 cc)

          a. Used off-label
          b. Inexpensive
       2. Ranibizumab (Lucentis, 0.5 mg in 0.05 cc)

          a. FDA-approved for monthly or prn
          b. ANCHOR and MARINA Studies: superior to observation or PDT 1
       3. Aflibercept (Eylea, 2 mg in 0.05 cc)

          a. FDA-approved for monthly injection and bimonthly maintenance
          b. VIEW1 and 2 Studies: non-inferior to Lucentis monthly

h. <u>OTHER INDICATIONS FOR OFF-LABEL INTRAVITREAL ANTI-VEFG (BEVACIZUMAB)</u>

    i. Chronic Central Serous Retinopathy
    ii. Choroidal or retinal vascular tumors
    iii. Choroidal neovascularization

       1. Myopic degeneration
       2. Presumed ocular histoplasmosis
       3. Choroidal rupture
       4. Angioid streaks
       5. Idiopathic

    iv. Iris Neovascularization
    v. Retinopathy of Prematurity,

       1. Dose: 0.625 mg in 0.025 cc
       2. Indication: zone 1, Stage 3 plus

i. <u>VITREO-MACULAR TRACTION</u>

    i. Intravitreal Ocriplasmin (Jetrea, 0.125 mg in 0.1 cc)

        1. Single application
        2. Contraindicated in eyes with loose lens zonules
        3. Adverse effects: lens subluxation, eye pain, ERG changes, etc.

3. Adverse Effects of Intravitreal Injection

Based on antiVEGF therapy among exudative AMD eyes

    i. Endophthalmitis: 0.09%
    ii. Chronic elevation in intraocular pressure (3 to 5%)
    iii. Uveitis 0.11%
    iv. Vitreous hemorrhage 0.23%
    v. Retinal tear or detachment (rare)
    vi. Acute transient elevation in intraocular pressure

        1. May accelerate progression of glaucoma in predisposing eyes

List of Abbreviations

AAO	American Academy of Ophthalmology
ACE	Angiotensin converting enzyme
AD	Autosomal dominant
AF	Autofluoresence
ANA	Anti-nuclear antibody
AP-ROP	Aggressive posterior retinopathy of prematurity
AR	Autosomal recessive
AREDS	Age-related Eye Disease Study
ARN	Acute retinal necrosis
AMD	Age-related macular degeneration
APMPPE	Acute posterior multifocal placoid pigment epitheliopathy
AZOOR	Acute zonal occult outer retinopathy
BARN	Bilateral acute retinal necrosis
BRAO	Branch retinal artery occlusion
BRVO	Branch retinal vein occlusion
BSS	Balanced saline solution
BW	Birth weight
CAR	Cancer associated retinopathy
CATT	Comparison of Age-related macular degeneration Treatment Trial
CHLA	Children's Hospital in Los Angeles
CME	Cystoid macular edema
CMT	Central macular thickness
CMV	Cytomegalovirus
CNVM	Choroidal neovascularization
CNS	Central nervous system

CPEO	Chronic progressive external ophthalmoplegia
CRAO	Central retinal artery occlusion
CRVO	Central retinal vein occlusion
CSCR	Central serous chorioretinopathy
CSF	Cerebrospinal fluid
CSME	Clinically significant macular edema
CT	Computerized tomography
DHA	Docosahexaenoic acid
DM	Diabetes mellitus
DME	Diabetic macular edema
DRS	Diabetic Retinopathy Study
DUSN	Diffuse unilateral sub-acute neuroretinitis
EBR	External beam radiation
EDI	Enhanced depth imaging mode
EOG	Electro-oculogram
ERG	Electroretinography or electroretinogram
ERM	Epiretinal membrane
ETDRS	Early Treatment of Diabetic Retinopathy Study
EVS	Endophthalmitis vitrectomy study
FA	Fluorescein angiography
FAZ	Foveal avascular zone
FDA	Food and Drug Administration
FEVR	Familial exudative vitreoretinopathy
ffERG	Full-field electroretinography
FTMH	Full-thickness macular hole
GA	Geographic atrophy
GCL	Ganglion cell layer
HSV	Herpes simplex virus
HZV	Herpes zoster virus
IAC	Intra-arterial chemotherapy
ICG	Indocyanine green dye
ILM	Internal limiting membrane
IMRT	Intensity-modulated Radiation Therapy
INL	Inner nuclear layer
IOFB	Intraocular foreign body
IOL	Intraocular lens implant
IOP	Intraocular pressure
IPL	Inner plexiform layer
IS/OS	Inner segment-outer segment junction

IV	Intravenous
IVC	Intravitreal chemotherapy
JIA	Juvenile idiopathic arthritis
KP	Keratic precipitates
K-pro	Keratoprosthesis
MA	Micro aneurysm
MAR	Melanoma associated retinopathy
MCP	Multifocal choroidal and pan uveitis
MEWDS	Multiple evanescent white dot syndrome
mfERG	Multifocal eletroretinography
MIC	Mean inhibitory concentration
MR	Mental retardation
MRI	Magnetic resonance imaging
MS	Multiple sclerosis
MSKCC	Memorial Sloan-Kettering Cancer Center
NFL	Nerve fiber layer
NV	Neovascularization
NV-AMD	Neovascular age-related macular degeneration
NVA	Neovascularization of the angle
NVD	Neovascularization of the disc
NVE	Neovascularization elsewhere
NVG	Neovascular glaucoma
NVI	Neovascularization of the iris
OAT	Ornithine aminotransferase
OCT	Optical coherence tomography
OIS	Ocular ischemic syndrome
ONL	Outer nuclear layer
OPL	Outer plexiform layer
PCV	Polypoidal Choroidal Vasculopathy
PDR	Proliferative diabetic retinopathy
PDT	Photodynamic therapy
PFO	Perfluorocarbon
PFV	Persistent fetal vasculature
PIC	Punctate inner choroiditis
PMA	Postmenstrual age
POHS	Presumed ocular histoplasmosis syndrome
PORN	Progressive outer retinal necrosis
PPD	Tuberculin skin test
PPV	Pars planar vitrectomy

PRP	Pan Retinal laser photocoagulation
PVD	Posterior vitreous detachment
PVR	Proliferative vitreoretinopathy
RA	Rheumatoid arthritis
RAP	Retinal angiomatous proliferation
RD	Retinal detachment
RF	Rheumatoid factor
RP	Retinitis pigmentosa
RPE	Retinal pigment epithelium
ROP	Retinopathy of prematurity
RVO	Retinal vein occlusion
SB	Scleral buckle
SDM	Subthreshold diode micropulse
SLE	Systemic Lupus Erythematosus
SO	Sympathetic ophthalmia
SRD	Serous retinal detachment
SUN	Standardization of Uveitis Nomenclature
TB	Tuberous sclerosis
TINU	Tubulo-interstitial nephritis and uveitis
TPA	Tissue plasminogen activator
TRD	Tractional retinal detachment
UBM	Ultrabiomicroscopy
UV	Ultraviolet
VEGF	Vascular endothelial growth factor
VF	Visual field
VH	Vitreous hemorrhage
VKH	Vogt-Koyanagi-Harada
VMT	Vitreomacular traction
XR	X-linked recessive

Index